PSYCHIATRIC
SYNDROMES
and
DRUG TREATMENT

PSYCHIATRIC SYNDROMES

and

DRUG TREATMENT

Nathan S. Kline, M.D.

Director, Rockland Research Institute
Clinical Professor of Psychiatry, Columbia University
Medical Director, Regent Hospital

Jules Angst, M.D.

Professor of Clinical Psychiatry, University of Zurich
Research Director, Department of Psychiatry, University of Zurich

New York • Jason Aronson • London

ISBN: 0–87668–379–0

Library of Congress Catalog Number: 79–51930

Manufactured in the United States of America

CONTENTS

PREFACE

In this volume we have presented a new and different approach to the subject of psychopharmacology. In the course of several long conversations we discovered that each of us as practicing clinicians and researchers had separately and individually evolved the same approach to decision making about the administration of psychotropic drugs to individual patients. We were strongly encouraged by the total agreement between us regarding the method we used to group patients, and again in respect to the choice of medications for each specific group. This information is easily communicated and it is in order to share these views, which we believe will be useful to others, that we have written this book. The division of psychiatric disorders into approximately fifty syndromes does result in some patients falling into the interstices. This, however, is true of any system of classification presently available. The classification by syndromes does seem to meet the reality more closely than does any other system.

The recommendations for treatment, including the dosages, are based primarily upon the experience of the authors. In many cases there are no controlled studies to demonstrate the validity of such decisions. In quite a number of instances the recommendations differ from those of the manufacturer. Our justification for this might be summed up in the statement "They only manufacture the drug; we treat the patients with it." In those instances where we have not had personal experience with the drug, the information is based on a search of the literature plus the advice of knowledgeable colleagues when it could be obtained. Appreciation is expressed to Prof. Heinz Lehmann of Montreal for his review and comments on parts of the manuscript. Acknowledgement is due also to Dr. Gaston Plantiff Loomis for his role in collating part of the data. The bibliographic, secretarial and other assistance of Anja Gubser of Zürich and Edna Robinson and Miriam Salzman of Orangeburg, N.Y. was invaluable.

As more information about the processes underlying psychiatric disorders becomes available, the syndromes should become more clearly defined. Because of the incomplete state of information about biochemical mechanisms of action, as well as only partial knowledge in respect to mode of pharmacological activity, we have decided to omit discussion of the pharmacology and biochemistry.

The creation of a new approach such as this is a most stimulating experience. We hope that the reader recognizes in his patients the same syndromes we identify and that the therapeutic responses he obtains are as satisfactory as our own.

Since the writing of this book was completed, a number of developments have come to our attention which require mention here:

1. The evidence that major tranquilizers produce tardive dyskinesia has continued to accumulate. A distinction should be made between (a) the dyskinesia which develops after the patient has been on high doses of medication but which disappears upon reduction of dosage or within six months of discontinuance, and (b) that which appears to be permanent. The former must be judged in terms of the usual side effect/therapeutic benefit evaluation. The latter, the permanent tardive dyskinesia, is much rarer and is another reason for not using medicine casually. It must be considered on a risk-benefit basis. While a number of studies have indicated lecithin to be of benefit, others have not. At present it is worth trying since no risk is involved. Considerable research is underway with the aim of finding a better corrective.

2. The recommendation we have made that low doses of major tranquilizers be substituted when there is evidence of tolerance or dependence on minor tranquilizers still stands. Tardive dyskinesia appears to be dose-related, and it is unlikely that it would occur with minimal doses. The possibility should be weighed against the

dangers of drug dependence or the devastation of the illness should there be tolerance with the minor tranquilizers.

3. Based on retrospective data there is some evidence that patients who receive lithium in addition to the major tranquilizers show much less tendency to develop tardive dyskinesia. This obviously has to be confirmed in prospective studies but there are theoretical reasons which would be compatible with such a finding. Certainly if the schizophrenia is of the recurring type described by Snezhnevsky, the concurrent use of lithium would be indicated.

4. There have been some claims that damage to kidney tubules occurs in some patients after prolonged use of lithium. At a major conference held in 1978 on all aspects of lithium, this subject was carefully reviewed. The meeting was a closed one and the proceedings will be published later this year as *Lithium: Controversies and Unresolved Issues*, published by Excerpta Medica. The editors are: Thomas B. Cooper, Samuel Gershon, Nathan S. Kline, and Mogens Schou. The same conclusion was reached at the International Group for the Study of Affective Disorders which met in Europe in 1979. Excerpts from the manuscripts presented at the 1978 Lithium Congress are being published in a Special Supplement by the *Archives of General Psychiatry*. The question was raised as to whether the conferees should make a recommendation on this score. The decision was that the data were inconclusive at the present time. There is some indication that patients who develop polydipsia and polyuria may be at greater risk, but even this is uncertain. Attention should be paid to future findings of research in this area.

5. Two important new drugs have emerged which may soon be available in the U.S., U.K., and Canada. One of these is deprenyl, marketed by Chinoin, Budapest under the trade name Jumex. The pressor amines in foods, such as tyramine, are inactivated by monoamine oxidase in the intestines, blood vessels, and tissue. Deprenyl selectively inhibits monoamine oxidase-B, whih deanimates benzylamines, but does not affect monoamine oxidase-A, which deanimates serotonin. Thus the drug is very useful in treating depression since it is a potent monoamine oxidase inhibitor (MAOI) but does not produce a "cheese" reaction so that dietary restrictions are not required. The second drug is piracetam, produced by U.C.B. in Belgium. It is marketed under a variety of proprietary names— Nootropil (South Africa), Nootropyl (France), Ideaxan (France),

and Normabrain (Germany). Piracetam may be the first member of a new class of drugs, a unique type of cerebral stimulant. There are reports of its usefulness in a variety of conditions characterized by reduced mental activity and impaired memory. Some research indicates that these functions also may be improved in relatively normal individuals.

This book is a syndrome approach to treatment. It can be used as an adjunct to the works on diagnosis, D.S.M. III and W.H.O. International Classification of Diseases.

Part I. General Principles of Psychopharmaceutical Treatment

WHY AND WHEN DRUG TREATMENT

If it is not absolutely necessary to *use* drugs, then it is absolutely necessary *not* to use drugs. This adaptation of one of Lord Acton's aphorisms expresses succinctly the most desirable attitude toward pharmacotherapy. Part of the normal human plight is to struggle out of depression, to bear the acid of anxiety, to withstand the pangs of remorse and the bites of guilt. All of these comprise part of the human condition and without them we would be less than, or certainly other than, human. We would also lack much of the world's great art, literature and music.

Problems arise when we attempt to define where "normal" merges into pathological. Even here, however, simple pathology is not necessarily an indication for treatment. The positive indications for treatment are the existence of a condition which (1) endangers life (the patient's or someone else's); (2) and/or produces severe and prolonged pain (which varies with individuals because of differences in pain thresholds); (3) and/or seriously interferes with productive capacity.

When one or more of these conditions exist, treatment *is* indicated. Mood swings, anxiety, and even auditory or visual hallucinations do not of themselves indicate a need for medical treatment unless they meet these criteria or constitute symptoms the patient wishes to be rid of.

UNNECESSARY DRUG TREATMENT

Not only should there be a clear indication for starting treatment but, once it has been started, there must be periodic evaluations as to whether medication should be continued. There is a great tendency to let well enough alone, so that if a patient is doing well there may be a strong reluctance to try reduced medication or to evaluate the advisability of discontinuance.

In the case of the anxiety syndromes, if dosage is above the minimal level, then, as a rule, medication should not be continued beyond two or three months. The major tranquilizers used in low doses do not act as rapidly nor are they as "satisfying" to the patient, yet they possess the advantage of not being habit-forming and also do not require escalation of dose since tolerance rarely develops. If it appears that the patient is suffering from chronic anxiety, then, after a month or two, there should be a gradual switchover from the minor to low doses of the major tranquilizer. Once this has been accomplished, the minor tranquilizer should be gradually withdrawn.

In the case of depressive syndromes, it is wise to allow the patient to continue on a substantial dose of medication for at least two months after remission of symptoms. At the end of this time, however, the medication should gradually be withdrawn. If it turns out that long-term maintenance is indicated, or if there is a tendency toward recurrence, then lithium should be gradually substituted for the antidepressant. There are cases, however, where lithium in combination with a very low dose of an antidepressant is the optimal treatment.

In the case of the schizophrenic syndromes, there is often the temptation to allow the patient to continue on the maximal dose to ensure that there will be no recurrence of symptoms. This possibility, however, can usually be handled by gradual withdrawal of medication with changes only every few months. Under conditions of recurrence a high dose should be reinstituted until the symptoms again disappear. The amount of medication should then be reduced to maintenance levels.

The use of antiparkinsonian drugs in combination with the major tranquilizers is fairly common. Care must be exercised since often these medications are continued indefinitely without good reason.

In a substantial number of cases, after a month or two the antiparkinsonian drug can gradually be withdrawn and the patient continued on the *major tranquilizer* without difficulty.

HOW TO HANDLE THE FAMILY

In almost every case there is a real ambivalence from the family toward the patient. At the very least the patient has produced a great deal of concern, often quite different from concern over physical diseases. Often the patient, the family, or both feel that they ought to have been able to prevent or at the very least to control and correct the psychological problems by providing more love, by being more strict or more lenient, or by explaining what has happened and why. This is probably in part because psychological disorders seem to be merely exaggerations of normal behavior, and there is no such clear-cut distinction as usually obtains between physical disease and physical health.

Some members of the family usually find the patient's behavior "threatening" in a variety of ways. Aside from fear of physical harm to others or harm to the patient, for either of which the family will be blamed, most so-called completely normal people *do* have a fear of becoming themselves mentally or emotionally disordered. When mental illness actually happens to a member of the family, all these anxieties and apprehensions are aroused. Under the circumstances, other family members may wish, for fear of being embarrassed, that the patient was out of the house or otherwise isolated from social contacts with people they know. Such feelings in turn often produce guilt, since one is not "supposed" to feel this way.

Nor is the patient usually blameless. The illness may be used as an occasion to vent long-felt grievances which have nothing to do with the illness; it is certainly not unknown for patients to exploit their illness for all sorts of secondary gain. The patient too often feels guilty that he is provoking an apparently unnecessary disturbance and is in danger of becoming a serious burden on the family. There is also, of course, the obvious fear that the illness is untreatable or that it will become progressively worse.

The first response on the part of both the patient and the family is usually denial. All sorts of aberrations of thought, feeling, and behavior are explained away in an effort to avoid the stigma, the cost, and the trauma of acknowledging a psychiatric disorder. The casual acquaintance or the treating physician when he first sees the patient is often amazed at the extent of the pathology. It can be erroneously concluded that the family is insensitive and unaware of the reality or even that the patient is dull in addition to being ill.

Once the illness has been acknowledged, there are a variety of reactions possible for both the patient and the family: overconcern, indifference (sometimes a continuance of the denial), or, in the best situations, normal concern with a realistic, helpful attitude. In almost every case the greatest need of the patient is for support. This is sometimes easier to subscribe to than to provide. Ordinary reassurance is not enough and often evidence must be provided over and over again that the family believes that the patient will recover.

This in turn entails certain obligations on the part of the treating physician. Not only the patient but usually members of the family as well are in need of explanation and reassurance. How and to what extent this is done obviously depends upon the individual family. There can be no set routine but probably a good general rule to follow is to provide only as much detail as requested and as much explanation as can be absorbed. There is certainly a minimum that the family should know, but in some cases the family much prefers to have the physician assume the fullest possible responsibility. Not to respect these wishes would be analogous to burdening a family with the details of a colon resection or prostatectomy when it serves no useful purpose. There are other cases where the family or one of its members is intensely and intelligently interested, and in such cases the explanation should not be too foreshortened. Often the degree of detail to be provided can be evaluated by determining how much information the family has already garnered by reading or through other means. At times the patient or family are reluctant to display their knowledge. Sometimes the physician can determine this only by asking the family how much they know about this or that aspect of the disease. Under this sort of inquiry the physician may discover that a great deal of information has been collected but that much of it is wrong. It is then his responsibility to sort out the known from the unknown and the correct from the incorrect.

One caution is to beware of the persistent questioner whose search is not for constructive proposals but for facts or opinions that can be used against the patient to intimidate and control or to provoke rejection by other members of the family. One way of identifying such individuals is that, given the opportunity, they usually seek confirmation of one or another of their preexisting prejudices. Even patients may fall into this category, although obviously to their ultimate disadvantage.

All of this means that, before providing such information and reassurance as the family appears to need, one should listen in order to best determine how much and in what form the family should be educated about the patient's condition.

DRUG USE AND ABUSE

> Oh, Doctor can you give me a pill to make me sleep. Oh, I'm working too hard and, oh, I'm worried about my marriage, and, oh, I'm worried about my job, and, oh, I can't stand what I think. Oh, give me a pill . . . .
> —Doris Lessing, *Briefing for a Descent into Hell*

Drug abuse is only one small part, a consequence and not a cause, of the upheaval in Western society. An attitude like the one depicted above does not produce the real problem but obviously is an attempt to escape from it. It is evidence of an inability to cope. Overconcern about drug use has produced not only a ridiculous but a frightening situation since, in order to discourage drug *abuse,* some people take seriously the idea that we ought to discourage drug *use* in general. As a result, many patients today are dangerously *un*medicated or *under*medicated and literally millions of suffering humans are deprived of the use of pharmaceutical agents which at the very least would make painful illnesses more bearable for them. As a consequence of well-intentioned but misdirected propaganda campaigns, more patients have died from not using drugs than have been "saved" by avoiding unnecessary ones.

Let us state at once that we are firmly opposed to legalization for general nonmedical use of opiates and support both legislative and enforcement procedures to control their abuse. As to cannabis, our knowledge of the effects is so limited that we would also oppose legalization for general use unless and until we know more about its physiological and psychological safety.

THE ROLE OF DRUGS IN TROUBLED TIMES

The worldwide disruption in value systems has resulted in the need by some for emotional analgesia. When stability returns to society and when the "narrative thread of existence" once more becomes viable, the demand for agents of escape and distortion will gradually decrease. Wars and depressions may be painful but they are not disruptive if there is a sense of meaning, an orientation in time, which is lacking today.

When our frame of reference is damaged or dismantled we solace ourselves as best we can with rampant consumerism, mystagogic cults, celebration of the sensate—and drug abuse—until some new and meaningful thrust carries us with it. The attempt of man to solve his problems pharmacologically is neither new nor unique. In each era we use the means at hand to attempt control of both our external and internal universes. Most cultures and civilizations have gone through an early period when there was appeasement of the spirits controlling the world whose goodwill could be obtained by offering up the first fruits of the season, by contributing various anatomical segments of livestock, captured enemies, or slaves, and even, on occasion, by sacrificing surplus neighbors. For half a millennium prayer was regarded as the choice method of dealing with otherwise insoluble problems. Within our own lifetime we have seen attempted sociopolitical solutions ranging from fascism to communism, from the old right to the new left. We have almost lived out an attempt to resolve all that is unresolvable through psychotherapy. The sociologist and anthropologist are now waiting in the wings to make their debut.

Panpharmaceas have never been more successful than any of the other panaceas. Yet because drugs do not solve all of life's problems is no reason to reject them in toto. The use of drugs, in fact, like art, music, and the dance, has always been with us in one form or another. There has probably never been a culture that did not at some stage use drugs, primarily as an integral part of religious and ritual functions. The turmoil of values and the lack of a coherent rational scenario in the external universe today has augmented the value of agents which can cut us off from this unsatisfactory actuality and help us to focus on "inner reality." This secular use of drugs is relatively new. Conditions favoring it have been present for the past few decades, but it was the introduction of the synthetic products of chemistry (and the refinement of natural products) that set the stage for today's problem. Within the past century the conviction has become almost universal that through chemistry we will eventually succeed in finding treatment for all medical disorders. The insistence that emotional and mental disorders are medical has naturally led to their inclusion as amenable to pharmacological management—and in fact there have been some brilliant successes.

In the broadest sense, of course, pharmacological agents are used virtually every day by every one of us. Whether they are sold, by prescription only or over the counter, or are contained in food as naturally occurring, semirefined, or synthetic agents does not gainsay their being drugs. Caffein, whether in coffee, tea, or soft drinks, has a well-defined set of pharmacological actions. There have been serious advocates of the theory that farming began in order to produce alcohol rather than mere food substances which could be obtained by hunting and gathering. Nicotine in the past five hundred years has had an interesting and checkered history.

When it is found that for certain conditions pharmacological agents are either not effective or that the side effects outweigh the benefits, most people will turn to new panaceas. There will still remain, however, many biological problems which in the end will require pharmacological solutions.

THE USE OF DRUGS FOR MEDICATION

The number of prescriptions written by physicians in private practice in the United States gives some idea of drug use. In 1960 the average patient received 5.7 prescriptions, an average which increased to 6.4 in 1970. Incidentally, in 1960 males received 4.6 prescriptions as contrasted with approximately 50 percent more (6.8) for females; the same proportion held in 1970, with 5.2 prescriptions for males and 7.5 for females. Over-the-counter sales averaged about $2 for ethical and $8 for proprietaries against $15 for prescriptions.

This use is actually quite conservative when one considers the advances in medicine and pharmacology. One hundred years ago we were abysmally ignorant about medications to treat most diseases.

Consider the effectiveness of drugs for high blood pressure, leprosy, pneumonia, schizophrenia, diabetes, depression, manic states, allergies, endocrine disorders, vitamin deficiencies, and malaria. Aspirin, discovered in 1899, has probably done more to control opiate consumption than have all the enforcement agencies in the world. Smallpox vaccination is less than a century old; adrenalin was first manufactured only seventy years ago. Thyroxine, insulin, chemical fumigators and insecticides, penicillin, vitamins B, B_2, A, and D, sulfonamides, antibiotics, and cortisone were all discovered, isolated, or applied clinically for the first time within our own lifetime. At least 20 percent of the population of the United States would be dead and another 20 percent maimed or crippled were it not for drugs discovered in this past century. Half of the people reading this book probably owe their health on at least one occasion to such medications. Even in the last twenty-five years there has been a quantum leap: from 12,000 pounds of penicillin in 1945 to over 3,000,000 pounds; from no streptomycin to 1,000,000 pounds a year; from nothing twenty years ago to nearly 2,000,000 pounds of psychopharmaceuticals today.

There obviously exist circumstances in which drugs are used to excess or needlessly, but resultant harm is minuscule compared with the damage resulting from failure to take medications when they are needed—or even to take adequate doses when they are prescribed.

One of the most apposite comments in this regard appeared in a letter sent to one of us by the father of a patient who refused medication and as a consequence had to be involuntarily hospitalized. He wrote: "All the publicity against the use of drugs has registered in the minds of some of those in need of treatment and has become a part of their thinking. It convinces them not to accept treatment when it is needed." For those of us in psychiatric practice, life is a continual struggle to get patients to accept and remain on the medications prescribed. In a variety of studies which have been done, the statistics clearly indicate that the rate of readmission to mental hospitals for patients who do not remain on medication is four times as great as for those patients who take drugs as prescribed.

Twenty years ago Kline and Brill (120) estimated the problem in terms of initial hospitalization and came to the conclusion that probably 80 percent of the patients then admitted to mental hospitals need not have been there had they been given appropriate medication in their own communities. Psychiatry has been particularly fouled up by the "I must do it by myself" myth. There are rare exceptions, but in most cases it makes as much sense to tell a diabetic "to pull himself together" and stop using insulin as it does to give this advice to a psychiatric patient. Willpower or even wish power is a poor substitute for digitalis—or a psychopharmaceutical—when it is indicated.

A great deal of this attitude arises from the indiscriminate trumpeting that our society is "overmedicated." It is no coincidence that the cries of alarm rarely come from those of us actually concerned with the treatment of patients. It certainly can be argued that we physicians have something to gain by the use of these drugs—most notably the improvement of our patients and the more adequate fulfillment of our responsibilities. The only people who stand to gain financially from such dire pronouncements are precisely those physicians who do *not* adequately medicate their patients—an omission that will usually result in the necessity for seeing them more frequently and over longer periods of time.

Side effects discourage use of a drug, so pharmaceutical companies tend to propose relatively low doses in the hope of avoiding such reactions; the physician, to be on the safe side, usually stays well below the maximum dose recommended by the pharmaceutical company and the patient then reduces or skips the amounts prescribed. It's a wonder so many patients do respond. Success in treatment is largely the result of prescribing adequate doses and insisting that the patient take the medication as ordered.

Even then we often fight a losing battle, and at times a few relapses are necessary to convince the patient that we know what we're talking about. Certainly there are things that can be done to simplify treatment: most, but not all, medications are as effective given once a day instead of in three or four doses; the body often compensates so that drugs against side effects (such as antiparkinsonian agents) can often be eliminated or reduced after the first month; reduction in dosage and eliminating of unneeded drugs should be tested for regularly. But it is the patient who unfortunately reduces medication prematurely, not so much to save money as to deny that he is really ill enough to require treatment.

WHEN AND HOW TO TERMINATE TREATMENT

Perhaps in the not too distant future there will be biochemical indices which can be measured in the blood or urine giving us an indication of whether or not medication should be continued. In the absence of such indices we are dependent on clinical experience. As a general rule it is probably best to discontinue medication gradually. Abrupt discontinuance of the minor tranquilizers can sometimes produce convulsions. Their sudden absence may also produce a craving for them which may trip off a drug dependence. Just as medication can be built up by increments of roughly 50 percent every week or two, so the minor tranquilizers can similarly be reduced by halving the dosage every week or two until the total amount is low enough to be discontinued without noticeable effect.

In respect to the antidepressants and the major tranquilizers, it is advisable to continue medication at full dosage or near full dosage for two to three months after symptoms have disappeared or are reduced to a therapeutically satisfactory minimum. At this point the same procedure should be followed, i.e., halving the dosage every two to three weeks in order to determine whether symptoms of the disorder will appear when the medication is lowered. In some cases it is advisable to wait even longer between reduction of dosage to determine whether evidence of the disorder will again become prominent. Obviously, should symptoms begin to reappear, the dosage should be again increased or an alternative medication provided.

Even after the patient is totally off all medications, it is the better part of judgment to have them return every three to six months for a one-year period. Often when symptoms begin to reappear the patient is reluctant to again enter into treatment; if he or she is discharged it is even more difficult to recommence treatment. If periodic checkup visits have been established as a routine, however, the process is much less traumatic.

Obviously in the case of the depressive syndromes, if there is a recurrence within the one-year period, or even before medications are completely discontinued, then the use of lithium should be given serious consideration. Under these circumstances a full regimen of antidepressant medications should be reinstituted at once and, as the patient begins to improve a second time, the lithium should be added.

In the case of patients with schizophrenic syndromes who need a maintenance dose, an analogy can be drawn to diabetes, hypothyroidism, or heart disease, as well as to other medical conditions in which maintenance doses of medication are necessary for the preservation of health.

Part II. The Syndromes: Psychopathology and Psychopharmacological Treatment

1. THE PRINCIPLES OF CLASSIFICATION BY SYNDROME

Categories, classifications, groupings are correct only insofar as they are useful. The use may be to systematize scientific knowledge (e.g., the chemical structure of psychotropic drugs) or to provide guides to treatment (e.g., dividing drugs according to their therapeutic effect); alternatively, the use may be cautionary (e.g., to protect against unwanted or dangerous side effects through a knowledge of mode of action). The number and nature of the categories is limited only by the needs or desires to answer one or another question.

How can we treat patients most effectively? The deceptively simple answer is: by giving the correct drugs to the appropriate patient.

Rather than describe each drug separately in great detail, it is obviously more convenient to lump together drugs with similar major therapeutic effect and then detail the minor differences between them. Some other feature may or may not coincide with the major principle of classification (therapeutic effect), e.g., the chemical structure, the pharmacological mode of action, the side effects. These alternate principles of structuring the data may be used secondarily but never at the cost of disrupting the classification based on therapeutic response.

Once classification has been made using a selected major principle (in our case, therapeutic effect), we may secondarily introduce a second principle such as mode of action or chemical structure. For instance, the therapeutic category might be "antidepressants"; if there is nothing further to be gained or if knowledge is lacking as to how to how to divide the antidepressants into those effective against endogenous depression and those useful against reactive depression, then we might wish to consider a subcategory based on mode of action or chemical structure (e.g., tricyclics vs. monoamine oxidase inhibitors).

Some confusion was introduced into the classification of psychotropic drugs early on by establishing therapeutic effect as the principle of classification but violating that principle by setting up one category, neuroleptics, based on the entirely different principle of side effects. Many more up-to-date systems have switched to "antipsychotics," a category not really satisfactory since the drugs are not limited to use in psychotics. Also, drugs used in treating some of the psychoses are not included. We have used the term *major tranquilizer* although this is not entirely satisfactory either, since tranquilization implies reducing agitation. The use of *ataraxia* and *ataractic* was never broadly accepted. The coining of a neologism would be even more confusing. Fortunately the use of whatever word we do use is clear from the context and we do list the specific drugs to which we make reference. Therefore, *antipsychotic, major tranquilizer,* and *neuroleptic* are used interchangeably.

When a drug can be placed in more than one category it gives rise to a pseudoproblem: at first it might appear contradictory to say, for instance, that certain phenothiazines should be categorized as both antipsychotic and antianxiety agents. But there is really no contradiction if the principle of classification is therapeutic effect. The prejudice in favor of classifying according to chemical structure shows itself here: no one would be disturbed if we listed phenothiazines as the primary category, with antipsychotic and antianxiety as subcategories. Another case in point is that of the monoamine oxidase inhibitors: these can be prescribed for phobias, compulsions, and certain kinds of dysphoria and anxiety, in addition to their more common use as antidepressants. (The differences among classificatory systems are illustrated in the table on the facing page.)

In this book we will try to specify which principles of classification are being used in our discussion of specific drugs. While it may seem that all of this discussion of categories, diagnostic groupings, and classification is a waste of time, it is at the very basis of any psychiatric discussion. As Panzetta (160) states:

Primary Principle of Classification	Further Subdivision According to Primary Principle of Classification	Secondary Principle of Classification	Tertiary Principle of Classification
Example			
I. (chemical structure) phenothiazine	aliphatic nonaliphatic	(psychological state) retarded psychosis agitated psychosis	
II. (mode of action) MAO inhibitor		(chemical structure) hydrazine nonhydrazine	(psychological state) agitated depression retarded depression
III. (psychological state) antidepressants	agitated depressions retarded depressions	(some specific drugs) doxepin amitriptyline protriptyline nortriptyline tranylcypramine	

The classification systems exert an enormous influence on our orientation to the diseased person and give us language with which to communicate with our colleagues, give us etiologic factors which guide our medical interventions, give us the orientation for our basic clinical and epidemiologic studies, and give us theoretical models within which we try to broaden our conceptual understanding.

Fortunately, these general principles hold true when we turn to the equally perplexing problem of diagnosis. There is, however, general dissatisfaction with all the proposed systems of diagnostic categories. One response to this state of affairs is the proposal that we simply abolish all categories except "mentally ill," a suggestion which would put us back about two hundred years. Bacon put it rather neatly: "Error is to be preferred to chaos."

An alternative principle of classification exists: instead of classifying diagnostic entities we can classify symptoms. In the one case we are faced with the dilemma that if patients are divided by diagnosis, not all schizophrenics, nor all depressions, nor all anxiety states require the same medication. But neither do symptoms work very well as the basis for prescribing. Not every patient with psychosomatic complaints needs the same treatment as every other.

In addition, with a different medication for almost every symptom, most patients would be prescribed a pharmacological galaxy.

Happily there does exist a rational basis for prescribing: a configuration of feeling, thinking, and behaving occurring together (*syn*) in time (*drome*) constitutes a *syndrome*. The presence of a particular syndrome rather than the diagnosis, as Richardson (179) states, "is, in effect a statement about what to do next in investigation or in treatment." This decision is the matter of primary concern to the therapist.

Our recognition of the use of syndromes as the basis for prescribing arose out of a series of conversations between the two authors of this volume. In a discussion of how we decide which drug to use, there was a simultaneous realization that our decisions are made on the basis of such syndromes rather than diagnostic categories or individual symptoms.

We are aware that such a categorizing of patients is incomplete, that the categories are not mutually exclusive and not always "reinsertable" into the system of diagnosis used for administrative purposes. The only strong reason for using this system is that it works better than any other approach. Nor is this necessarily a bad thing. Panzetta concludes his paper (160) with the following paragraph:

Psychiatric Identity. The confusion of identity that psychiatry is now experiencing is, in my estimation, a scientifically healthy process. To put it into the terms used in this paper, the turmoil is a reflection of the inadequacy (both conceptual and practical) of our discipline's nosology. The turmoil will lead us to newer definitions, newer perspectives, and hopefully to a more valid level of communication with one another. For the time being it will be painful. But patients and their problems will not disappear just because our identity may be in a state of redefinition. They will keep us on a track that demands interventional relevance, communicational clarity, and practicality.

2. SCHIZOPHRENIC SYNDROMES

2.1. Passive paranoid schizophrenic syndrome

Psychopathology.   The syndrome is characterized by ideas of reference so that the patient is inclined to interpret ordinary facts and ordinary reactions of other people in a delusional autistic way. Typical are delusions of persecution, delusions of influence, and delusions of reference connected with a special feeling which attaches great importance to what are actually insignificant experiences. The patient may develop (a) feelings of being observed and (b) feelings that his thoughts are being broadcast so that everyone knows what he is thinking. His answers about who is doing the watching and why are vague, and his response to imagined persecutions is inappropriate since more or less passive—he has no intention of doing anything to alter this state of affairs and no active plans to protect himself. The syndrome is usually characterized by a reasonably good social adaptation. The patient is often able to hold a job or care for a home, talks reasonably and logically, and is not severely disturbed. There may, however, be frequent job changes to avoid persecution. The syndrome occurs quite frequently and is often not obvious to others.

Pharmacological treatment.   Give nonsedative major tranquilizers. Depot preparations, such as fluphenazine-decanoate, fluanxoldecanoate, and fluspirilene i.m., or the new oral long-acting preparations such as penfluridol, are especially indicated. The patient usually does not feel sick and is not inclined to take drugs. Therefore it is better to inject the drug or to use a preparation which can be given orally once a week.

Drugs indicated*:

Primary:	(86)	Perphenazine
		Perphenazine enanthate
	(47)	Fluphenazine dihydrochloride
	(46)	Fluphenazine decanoate
	(48)	Fluphenazine enanthate
	(7)	Butaperazine
	(123)	Thiopropazate
	(130)	Trifluoperazine
	(95)	Prochlorperazine
	(4)	Acetophenazine
	(9)	Carphenazine
	(125)	Thioridazine
	(93)	Piperacetazine
	(65)	Mesoridazine
	(100)	Propericiazine
	(191)	Flupenthixol
		Flupenthixol decanoate
	(243)	Thiothixene
	(621)	Haloperidol
	(633)	Trifluperidol
	(925)	Pimozide
	(199)	Clozapine

* Compound number and generic name according to Usdin and Efron (229a). The listing includes drugs on the market in all 3 countries (U.S.A., Canada and U.K.). In actual practice it is by far the best usage to be very familiar with a few drugs in each category and to use these first. If they fail to produce the desired results then one of the listed alternatives should be tried.

In combination with an antidepressant:

(156)	Amitriptyline
(245)	Trimepramine
(227)	Opipramol
(187)	Doxepin
(206)	Imipramine
(165)	Chlorimipramine (clomipramine)
(223)	Nortriptyline
(182)	Desipramine
(184)	Dibenzepin
(171)	Clofepramine (lopramine)
(164)	Carpipramine
(162)	Butriptyline
(236)	Protriptyline
(235)	Prothiaden
	Viloxazine
(1252)	Maprotiline (ludiomil)
	Mianserine
(1259)	Tofenacine
(776)	Iproniazid
(777)	Isocarboxazide
(867)	Nialamide
(1165)	Phenelzine
(397)	Iprindol
(994)	Trazodone
	Nomifensin
(1192)	Tranylcypromine
	L-tryptophan combined with pyridoxin and ascorbic acid
(156)	Amitriptyline combined with
(86)	Perphenazine
(156)	Amitriptyline combine with
(523)	Chlordiazepoxide
(47)	Fluphenazinedihydrochloride combined with
(223)	Nortriptyline
(1192)	Tranylcypromine(10 mg)combined with
(130)	Trifluoperzine (1 mg)

2.2. Florid paranoid agitated syndrome

Psychopathology. The syndrome is characterized by a delusional mood with a flood of productive psychotic symptoms such as hallucinations (mainly voices); they repeat aloud the patient's thoughts and may comment upon them; the voices are frequently accusatory, make nasty comments, or give uncongenial orders against the patient's wishes. The patient may feel that things are put into his mind and at other times that his thoughts are "snatched" away so that his mind suddenly goes blank. At times the feeling exists that someone or something other than himself is controlling his actions. As a consequence, the patient is agitated and anxious. His thinking is illogical, his speech sometimes incoherent. Communication is severely disturbed to a point where it is usually obvious to other people because the patient may be reacting to voices and even speaking to them.

Pharmacological treatment. The syndrome has to be treated by sedative major tranquilizers, for instance, chlorpromazine, chlorprothixene, clozapine, clopenthixol, and clotiapine, or with a combination of levomepromazine with a nonsedative major tranquilizer.

Drugs indicated:

Primary:	(98)	Promazine
	(20)	Chlorpromazine
	(132)	Trifluperazine
	(86)	Perphenazine
		Perphenazine enanthate
	(47)	Fluphenazine dihydrochloride
	(46)	Fluphenazine decanoate
	(48)	Fluphenazine enanthate
	(7)	Butaperazine
	(123)	Thiopropazate
	(130)	Trifluoperazine
	(95)	Prochlorperazine
	(4)	Acetophenazine
	(9)	Carphenazine
	(93)	Piperacetazine

(168)	Chlorprothixene
(173)	Clopenthixol
(621)	Haloperidol
(608)	Benperidol
(753)	Fluspirilene
(909)	Penfluridol
(199)	Clozapine
(318)	Reserpine

Secondary: none

2.3. Systematic paranoid syndrome

Psychopathology. The clinical picture is very clear but also very rare. The patient is often not recognized as mentally ill and does not feel ill either. His personality is very well preserved except for a circumscribed delusional area. The delusional system is very coherent, systematic, and logical. The delusions are frequently based on a single misinterpreted experience, or perhaps a series of such experiences. The patient speaks logically, easily convinces others, is inclined to fight for his convictions, and if necessary goes to court. Any discussions about his delusions are fruitless since he feels himself irrefutable.

Pharmacological treatment. The patient does not feel sick and does not want to be treated. In most cases it is impossible to get the patient to accept psychotropic drugs. Sometimes it is possible to give a sedative major tranquilizer instead of an ordinary hypnotic in the evening. The treatment has to be a long-term one over months because the whole process is a chronic one. If the patient is willing to take medication, those especially indicated are nonstimulant, nonsedative major tranquilizers such as butyrophenones, thioridazine, perphenazine, prochlorperazine, fluphenazine decanoate, and flupenthixol decanoate.

Drugs indicated:

Primary: (86) Perphenazine
                            Perphenazine enanthate

(47)	Fluphenazine dihydrochloride
(46)	Fluphenazine decanoate
(48)	Fluphenazine enanthate
(7)	Butaperazine
(123)	Thiopropazate
(130)	Trifluoperazine
(95)	Prochlorperazine
(4)	Acetophenazine
(9)	Carphenazine
(125)	Thioridazine
(93)	Piperacetazine
(65)	Mesoridazine
(100)	Propericiazine
(173)	Clopenthixol
(191)	Flupenthixol
	Flupenthixol decanoate
(243)	Thiothixene
(621)	Haloperidol
(633)	Trifluperidol
(925)	Pimozide
(753)	Fluspirilene
(909)	Penfluridol
(199)	Clozapine

Secondary:	(20)	Chlorpromazine
	(132)	Triflupromazine
	(168)	Chlorprothixene

2.4. Catatonic schizophrenic syndrome

Psychopathology. The picture is characterized by psychomotor inhibition, as well as inhibited speech, behavior, thinking, drive, and spontaneity. In severe cases we find a stupor with mutism and cataleptic symptoms. Very often the patient is blocked by a high level of inner anxiety. This may express itself in stereotypes of speech and behavior. The pathological inhibition can occasionally turn itself over into sudden outbursts, irrational dangerous acting out (catatonic raptus) with blind, indiscriminant aggression or impulsive suicidal attempts. These conditions are very dangerous.

Pharmacological treatment.   Antipsychotic drugs are often ineffective. Very strong nonsedative major tranquilizers are indicated, sometimes in combination with tricyclic antidepressants or small doses of MAOIs. (We use thiopropazate + chlorphencyclan [Vesitan] or sometimes even a sedative major tranquilizer like clozapine.) If the condition doesn't change within a few days, one should not hesitate to apply ECT, which is still the most effective method for rapid treatment of catatonic states.

Drugs indicated:

Primary:	(20)	Chlorpromazine
	(132)	Triflupromazine
	(86)	Perphenazine
		Perphenazine enanthate
	(47)	Fluphenazine dihydrochloride
	(46)	Fluphenazine decanoate
	(48)	Fluphenazine enanthate
	(7)	Butaperazine
	(123)	Thiopropazate
	(130)	Trifluoperazine
	(95)	Prochlorperazine
	(4)	Acetophenazine
	(9)	Carphenazine
	(125)	Thioridazine
	(93)	Piperacetazine
	(65)	Mesoridazine
	(100)	Propericiazine
	(173)	Clopenthixol
	(191)	Flupenthixol
		Flupenthixol decanoate
	(243)	Thiothixene
	(621)	Haloperidol
	(633)	Trifluperidol
	(608)	Benperidol
	(925)	Pimozide
	(753)	Fluspirilene
	(909)	Penfluridol
	(199)	Clozapine
	(318)	Reserpine

In combination with a major tranquilizer:

(156)	Amitriptyline
(245)	Trimepramine
(227)	Opipramol
(187)	Doxepin
(206)	Imipramine
(165)	Chlorimipramine (clomipramine)
(223)	Nortriptyline
(182)	Desipramine
(184)	Dibenzepin
(171)	Clofepramine (lopramine)
(264)	Carpipramine
(162)	Butriptyline
(236)	Protriptyline
(235)	Prothiaden
(1252)	Maprotiline
	Mianserine
(1259)	Tofenacine
(776)	Iproniazid
(777)	Isocarboxazide
(867)	Nialamide
(1165)	Phenelzine
(1192)	Tranylcypromine
(397)	Iprindol
(994)	Trazodone
	Nomifensin
	L-tryptophan combined with pyridoxin and ascorbic acid
(156)	Amitriptyline combined with
(86)	Perphenazine
(156)	Amitriptyline combined with
(523)	Chlordiazepoxide
(47)	Fluphenazine dihydrochloride combined with
(223)	Nortriptyline
(1192)	Tranylcypromine (10 mg) combined with
(130)	Trifluoperazine (1 mg)

Secondary: (98) Promazine
         (168) Chlorprothixene

2.5. Simple schizophrenic syndrome

Psychopathology. The picture is characterized by very bland symptoms, flatness of affect, disturbance of contact, autistic modes of thinking and behavior, occasional complaints of depressed mood, feelings of inferiority, and inhibitions. However, in spite of these symptoms the patient doesn't appear to be depressed. He shows a loss of interest and a shift to bizarre autistic activities. The thinking is often deficient, occasionally incoherent and blocked. Loose associations, social withdrawal, and loss of ego boundaries are also characteristic of the syndrome.

Pharmacological treatment. The clinical picture is chronic and usually not influenced by pharmacotherapy. One can try a long-term treatment with such medications as carpipramine or thiothixene.

Drugs indicated:

    Primary: (86) Perphenazine
                    Perphenazine enanthate
           (47) Fluphenazine dihydrochloride
           (46) Fluphenazine decanoate
           (48) Fluphenazine enanthate
             (7) Butaperazine
          (123) Thiopropazate
          (130) Trifluoperazine
          (95) Prochlorperazine
            (4) Acetophenazine
            (9) Carphenazine
          (125) Thioridazine
          (93) Piperacetazine
          (65) Mesoridazine
         (100) Propericiazine
         (191) Flupenthixol
                    Flupenthixol decanoate

(243)	Thiothixene
(621)	Haloperidol
(633)	Trifluperidol
(925)	Pimozide
(199)	Clozapine

Secondary: (168) Chlorprothixene

2.6. Hebephrenic schizophrenic syndrome

Psychopathology. The psychopathology is unsystematic and characterized by silly and inappropriate behavior, inadequacy of affect, shallow affect, inadequate or even compulsive laughing, defective and awkward motor activity, loss of distance recognition, and at times motor agitation. Thought disorders and hallucinations or delusions may be present. The picture should not be confused with a manic state; the affect may be very similar but the content of the thoughts is not congruent with the mood.

Pharmacological treatment. Sedative major tranquilizers: clozapine, clopenthixol, chlorpromazine.

Drugs indicated:

Primary:
(86)	Perphenazine
	Perphenazine enanthate
(47)	Fluphenazine dihydrochloride
(46)	Fluphenazine decanoate
(48)	Fluphenazine enanthate
(7)	Butaperazine
(123)	Thiopropazate
(130)	Trifluoperazine
(95)	Prochlorperazine
(4)	Acetophenazine
(9)	Carphenazine
(125)	Thioridazine
(93)	Piperacetazine
(65)	Mesoridazine
(100)	Propericiazine
(168)	Chlorprothixene

(173) Clopenthixol
(191) Flupenthixol
        Flupenthixol decanoate
(243) Thiothixene
(621) Haloperidol
(753) Fluspirilene
(909) Penfluridol
(199) Clozapine
(318) Reserpine

Secondary: (20) Chlorpromazine
              (132) Triflupromazine

2.7. Schizophrenic withdrawal syndrome

Psychopathology. The clinical picture is a chronic residual state following an active schizophrenic process and characterized by severe lack of motivation, interest, and activity. The patient shows no need for social contact, is highly autistic and withdrawn, and may neglect himself without concern. He has lost all affective responsiveness and cannot be stimulated by others, nor is he very much affected by external events.

Pharmacological treatment. The chronic withdrawn schizophrenic syndrome is highly resistant to therapy. When pharmacological treatment is applied it has to last for months. Avoid sedative major tranquilizers. Try thiothixene, carpipramine, perphenazine plus amitriptyline (Triavil, Etrafon) or combine a nonsedative major tranquilizer with a tricyclic antidepressant or an MAOI.

Drugs indicated:

Primary: (86) Perphenazine
                    Perphenazine enanthate
             (47) Fluphenazine dihydrochloride
             (46) Fluphenazine decanoate
             (48) Fluphenazine enanthate
              (7) Butaperazine
            (123) Thiopropazate

(130) Trifluoperazine
(95) Prochlorperazine
(4) Acetophenazine
(9) Carphenazine
(125) Thioridazine
(93) Piperacetazine
(65) Mesoridazine
(100) Propericiazine
(168) Chlorprothixene
(191) Flupenthixol
      Flupenthixol decanoate
(243) Thiothixene
(621) Haloperidol
(633) Trifluperidol
(925) Pimozide
(199) Clozapine

In combination with a major tranquilizer:

(156) Amitriptyline
(245) Trimepramine
(227) Opipramol
(187) Doxepin
(206) Imipramine
(165) Chlorimipramine (clomipramine)
(223) Nortriptyline
(182) Desipramine
(184) Dibenzepin
(171) Clofepramine (lopramine)
(164) Carpipramine
(162) Butriptyline
(236) Protriptyline
(235) Prothiaden
      Viloxazine
(1252) Maprotiline
      Mianserine
(1259) Tofenacine
(776) Iproniazid
(777) Isocarboxazide

(867)   Nialamide
(1165)   Phenelzine
(1192)   Tranylcypromine
(397)   Iprindol
(994)   Trazodone
       Nomifensin
       L-tryptophan combined with
       pyridoxin and ascorbic acid
(156)   Amitriptyline combined with
(86)   Perphenazine
(156)   Amitriptyline combined with
(523)   Chlordiazepoxide
(47)   Fluphenazine dihydrochloride combined with
(223)   Nortriptyline
(1192)   Tranylcypromine (10 mg) combined with
(130)   Trifluoperazine (1 mg)

3. SCHIZOAFFECTIVE SYNDROMES

3.1. Manic-schizophrenic syndrome

Psychopathology. The patient is overactive; thinking is accelerated; pressure of speech is evident. Thinking is not characterized by a flight of ideas (as in the pure manic) but is incoherent or at least illogical. Usually there is no euphoria. Eventual the patient manifests delusions of grandeur or ideas of persecution or jealousy. His mood is irritable, dysphoric, tense, sometimes hostile, and occasionally ecstatic. He shows increased initiative and spontaneity, as well as logorrhea.

Pharmacological treatment. The same as for mania.

Drugs indicated:

Primary:	(20)	Chlorpromazine
	(132)	Triflupromazine
	(86)	Perphenazine
		Perphenazine enanthate
	(47)	Fluphenazine dihydrochloride
	(46)	Fluphenazine decanoate
	(48)	Fluphenazine enanthate
	(7)	Butaperazine
	(123)	Thiopropazate
	(130)	Trifluoperazine
	(95)	Prochloperazine
	(4)	Acetophenazine
	(9)	Carphenazine
	(93)	Piperacetazine
	(173)	Clopenthixol
	(621)	Haloperidol
	(753)	Fluspirilene
	(909)	Penfluridol
	(199)	Clozapine
	(318)	Reserpine
	(1552)	Lithium (prophylaxis)
Secondary:	(608)	Benperidol

3.2. Depressive-schizophrenic syndrome

Psychopathology. The clinical picture is characterized by a combination of depressive syndrome on the one hand and catatonic or
paranoid symptoms on the other. Usually the patient is inhibited,
retarded, restricted, and blocked, but his claimed depression does
not move the heart of the observer. The patient is more stiff than
depressed, more autistic than appealing for sympathy. He may show
symptoms of derealization and of illogical thinking with paralogia

and incoherence. Delusions of persecution, delusions of reference, or grotesque hypochondriasis may occur.

Pharmacological treatment   It is correct to combine a major tranquilizer with a tricyclic antidepressant or to give carpipramine or thiothixene.

Drugs indicated:

Primary: (86)   Perphenazine
                    Perphenazine enanthate
              (47)   Fluphenazine dihydrochloride
              (46)   Fluphenazine decanoate
              (48)   Fluphenazine enanthate
               (7)   Butaperazine
             (123)   Thiopropazate
             (130)   Trifluoperazine
              (95)   Prochlorperazine
               (4)   Acetophenazine
               (9)   Carphenazine
             (125)   Thioridazine
              (93)   Piperacetazine
              (65)   Mesoridazine
             (100)   Propericiazine
             (168)   Chlorprothixene
             (191)   Flupenthixol
             (243)   Thiothixene
             (621)   Haloperidol
             (633)   Trifluperidol
             (925)   Pimozide

In combination with a major tranquilizer:

             (156)   Amitriptyline
             (245)   Trimepramine

(227)   Opipramol
(187)   Doxepin
(206)   Imipramine
(165)   Chlorimipramine (clomipramine)
(223)   Nortriptyline
(182)   Desipramine
(184)   Dibenzepin
(171)   Clofepramine (lopramine)
(164)   Carpipramine
(162)   Butriptyline
(236)   Protriptyline
(235)   Prothiaden
        Viloxazine
(1252)   Maprotiline (ludiomil)
        Mianserine
(1259)   Tofenacine
(776)   Iproniazid
(777)   Isocarboxazide
(867)   Nialamide
(1165)   Phenelzine
(1192)   Tranylcypromine
(397)   Iprindol
(994)   Trazodone
        Nomifensin
        L-tryptophan combined with
        pyridoxin and ascorbic acid
(156)   Amitriptyline combined with
(86)   Perphenazine
(156)   Amitriptyline combined with
(523)   Chlordiazepoxide
(47)   Fluphenazine dihydrochloride combined
        with
(223)   Nortriptyline

(1192)   Tranylcypromine (10 mg) combined with
(130)   Trifluoperazine (1 mg)

4. AFFECTIVE SYNDROMES

4.1. Retarded depressive syndrome

Psychopathology. The patient complains of reduced capacity for enjoyment, loss of interest in work and family, reduced productivity, and disorders of attention and immediate memory. Thinking is inhibited, retarded, restricted, or even blocked. Appearance is depressed, hopeless, and sometimes anxious, and the patient complains of inner restlessness or of fatigue and lack of drive and energy. Thought is heavily loaded with depressive content. Guilt feelings or delusions of guilt, feelings of impoverishment, or delusions may be present. At times there is suffering from pressure in the head and throat. Vital feelings are disturbed. Characteristic also are diurnal fluctuations of symptoms, in which the patient feels worse in the morning. Usually there is early morning awakening and loss of appetite for both food and sexual activity. Suicidal tendencies must be looked for. Autonomic symptoms include constipation and dryness of the mouth. In severe cases, the condition progresses to stupor with complete blockage of speech and motor activity.

Pharmacological treatment. The patient has to be treated with tricyclic antidepressants in sufficiently high daily dosages (150 or more mg) or with MAOIs in similarly adequate amounts for at least three to four weeks. In resistant cases the use of an MAOI such as tranylcypromine combined with a suitable tricyclic may be needed.

If the patient is already on tricyclics a very low dose of the MAOI should be used initially and then gradually increased every few days up to a full dose or until the patient responds. Too rapid an increase may cause drop in blood pressure or other side effects. MAOIs may be introduced and increased more rapidly and safely with patients on tricyclics than may tricyclics with patients already on MAOIs.

In cases where there is sensitivity to other agents or where the patient is reluctant to use synthetic chemicals, tryptophane combined with nicotinamide and ascorbic acid may be adequate in doses of 500 mg of tryptophane (from 6 to 18/day). The tryptophane combination added to an MAOI may speed up the reaction. In severe cases or where there is great immediate danger of suicide consider the use of unilateral ECT.

Drugs indicated:

Primary:	(125)	Thioridazine
	(65)	Mesoridazine
	(168)	Chlorprothixene
	(243)	Thiothixene
	(156)	Amitriptyline
	(245)	Trimepramine
	(227)	Opipramol
	(187)	Doxepin
	(206)	Imipramine
	(165)	Chlorimipramine (clomipramine)
	(223)	Nortriptyline
	(182)	Desipramine
	(184)	Dibenzepin
	(171)	Clofepramine (lopramine)
	(164)	Carpipramine
	(162)	Butriptyline
	(236)	Protriptyline
	(235)	Prothiaden
		Viloxazine
	(1252)	Maprotiline (ludiomil)
		Mianserine
	(1259)	Tofenacine
	(776)	Iproniazid
	(777)	Isocarboxazide

    (867)   Nialamide
  (1165)   Phenelzine
  (1192)   Tranylcypromine
    (397)   Irpindol
    (994)   Trazodone
            Nomifensin
            L-tryptophan combined with
            pyridoxin and ascorbic acid
    (156)   Amitriptyline combined with
     (86)   Perphenazine
    (156)   Amitriptyline combined with
    (523)   Chlordiazepoxide
     (47)   Fluphenazine dihydrochloride combined
            with
    (223)   Nortriptyline
  (1192)   Tranylcypromine (10 mg) combined with
    (130)   Trifluoperazine (1 mg)
  (1552)   Lithium (prophylaxis)

Secondary: (100)   Propericiazine
    (191)   Flupenthixol
  (1098)   Dextroamphetamine
  (1147)   Methamphetamine
            Methylphenidate
    (931)   Piperadrol

Not in combination with tricyclics

  (1147)   Methamphetamine combined with
    (563)   Amobarbital
  (1147)   Methamphetamine combined with
            Phenobarbital-Na
  (1098)   Dextroamphetamine combined with
    (563)   Amobarbital

4.2. Agitated depressive syndrome

Psychopathology. The patient feels hopeless, desperate, and anxious suffering from agitation, motor restlessness, sleep disturbances, and lack of concentration. He is full of complaints, constantly appealing to others for help. Delusions of poverty, guilt, or hypochondriasis are frequently present, and the need for increased contact leads to his clinging to others in his anxiety. Diurnal rhythm is such that he may show improvement in the evening.

Pharmacological treatment.   This type of patient is difficult to treat. He has first of all to be sedated by an effective minor tranquilizer such as diazepam in combination with a sedative tricyclic antidepressant (amitriptyline, doxepin). In some cases levomepromazine can be used. If suicidal ideas are expressed they should be taken seriously and may indicate the need for hospitalization. Once again adequate doses of antidepressants for adequate periods of time are required. Combined tricyclic-phenothiazines (e.g., amitriptyline and perphenazine) may be useful.

Drugs indicated:

Primary:	(156)	Amitriptyline
	(245)	Trimepramine
	(227)	Opipramol
	(187)	Doxepin
	(206)	Imipramine
	(165)	Chlorimipramine (clomipramine)
	(223)	Nortriptyline
	(182)	Desipramine
	(184)	Dibenzepin
	(171)	Clofepramine (lopramine)
	(164)	Carpipramine
	(162)	Butriptyline
	(236)	Protriptyline
	(235)	Prothiaden
		Viloxazine
	(1252)	Ludiomil
		Mianserine
	(1259)	Tofenacine
	(397)	Iprindol
	(994)	Trazodone
		Nomifensin
		L-tryptophan combined with

	pyridoxin and ascorbic acid
(156)	Amitriptyline combined with
(86)	Perphenazine
(156)	Amitriptyline combined with
(523)	Chlordiazepoxide
(47)	Fluphenazine dihydrochloride combined with
(223)	Nortriptyline
(1552)	Lithium (prophylaxis)

Secondary:

(86)	Perphenazine
(47)	Fluphenazine dihydrochloride
(7)	Butaperazine
(123)	Thiopropazate
(130)	Trifluoperazine
(95)	Prochlorperazine
(4)	Acetophenazine
(9)	Carphenazine
(93)	Piperacetazine
(100)	Propericiazine
(173)	Clopenthixol
(621)	Haloperidol
(199)	Clozapine
(522)	Chlorazepate
(523)	Chlordiazepoxide
(528)	Diazepam
(533)	Lorazepam
(534)	Medazepam
(538)	Oxazepam
(1446)	Meprobamate
(768)	Hydroxyzine
	Hydroxyzine pamoate
(1470)	Methylpentynol
(1447)	Methylpentynol carbamate
(1104)	Benzoctamine
(704)	Chlormethazanone
(938)	Prothipendyl
(1361)	Methocarbamol
(1451)	Tybamate

(1212)   Benactyzine
(1371)   Phenaglycodol
(1242)   Captodiame
(1244)   Diphenhydramine

Combinations (see table, § **14**)

4.3. Affective hypochondriacal syndrome

Psychopathology.   The affective hypochondriacal patient always observes himself more carefully than the normal individual. He worries about his physical or mental condition with frequent concentration on his bowels, his constipation, his autonomic functions, on any paresthesias, dryness of the mouth, and so on. His hypochondriacal anxiety may increase to the point of a delusion that he is suffering from cancer or some other incurable disease. The patient insists upon being examined by many different doctors and in general is very unstable. He is full of complaints, anxiety, and hopelessness. His thinking is almost entirely restricted to bodily functions.

Pharmacological treatment.   Because he observes himself so carefully, the patient is likely to concentrate mainly on the autonomic side effects of the drug if an antidepressant is given. Start with a mild sedative tricyclic antidepressant or a combination of antidepressant with a minor tranquilizer: opipramol or some other minor tranquilizer in combination with amitriptyline in low dosages or with an MAOI. Avoid if possible autonomic side effects since they are apt to set up a vicious circle. Treat the patient over a period of weeks with the same drugs, disregarding the patient's very likely demands for a change every day or two. He is also likely to take the tablets irregularly because he is frightened that they may be harmful and suspects that the doctor may not have recognized the severe physical illness behind the complaints.

Drugs indicated:

   Primary: (156)   Amitripytyline
                  (245)   Trimipramine
                  (227)   Opipramol

(187)   Doxepin
(206)   Imipramine
(165)   Chlorimipramine (clomipramine)
(223)   Nortriptyline
(182)   Desipramine
(184)   Dibenzepin
(171)   Clofepramine (lopramine)
(164)   Carpipramine
(162)   Butriptyline
(236)   Protriptyline
(235)   Prothiaden
        Viloxazine
(1252) Maprotiline
        Mianserine
(1259) Tofenacine
(776)   Iproniazid
(777)   Isocarboxazide
(867)   Nialamide
(1165) Phenelzine
(1192) Tranylcypromine
(397)   Iprindol
(994)   Trazodone
        Nomifensin
        L-tryptophan combined with
        pyridoxin and ascorbic acid
(156)   Amitriptyline combined with
(86)   Perphenazine
(156)   Amitriptyline combined with
(523)   Chlordiazepoxide
(47)   Fluphenazine dihydrochloride combined
        with
(223)   Nortriptyline
(1192) Tranylcypromine (10 mg) combined with
(130)   Trifluoperazine (1 mg)
(1552) Lithium (prophylaxis)

Secondary: (20)   Chlorpromazine
               (132) Triflupromazine

(100)	Propericiazine
(522)	Chlorazepate
(523)	Chlordiazepoxide
(528)	Diazepam
(533)	Lorazepam
(534)	Medazepam
(538)	Oxazepam
(1446)	Meprobamate
(768)	Hydroxyzine
	Hydroxyzine pamoate
(1470)	Methylpentynol
(1447)	Methylpentynol carbamate
(1104)	Benzoctamine
(704)	Chlormethazanone
(938)	Prothipendyl
(1361)	Methocarbamol
(1451)	Tybamate
(1212)	Benactyzine
(1371)	Phenaglycodol
(1242)	Captodiame
(1244)	Diphenhydramine

Combinations (see table, § **14**)

4.4. Depressed obsessive-compulsive syndrome

Psychopathology The patient suffers from a clear-cut depressive state, most frequently of the retarded type, but additionally he suffers from obsessive thoughts, compulsive impulses, and actions. In contrast to an obsessive-compulsive neurosis these symptoms increase or decrease in accord with fluctuations in the depth of the depressive state.

Pharmacological treatment. The prognosis is not worse than that of other depressive syndromes, and the treatment should be aimed at the dominant retardation or agitation. There are no drugs with a proven particular effect on obsessive-compulsive symptoms although MAOIs have been claimed to be effective at times. Sometimes a minor tranquilizer or low dosages of a major tranquilizer may be useful.

Drugs indicated:

Primary:	(156)	Amitriptyline
	(245)	Trimepramine
	(227)	Opipramol
	(187)	Doxepin
	(206)	Imipramine
	(165)	Chlorimipramine (clomipramine)
	(223)	Nortriptyline
	(182)	Desipramine
	(184)	Dibenzepin
	(171)	Clofepramine (lopramine)
	(164)	Carpipramine
	(162)	Butriptyline
	(236)	Protriptyline
	(235)	Prothiaden
		Viloxazine
	(1252)	Maprotiline
		Mianserine
	(1259)	Tofenacine
	(776)	Iproniazid
	(777)	Isocarboxazide
	(867)	Nialamide
	(1165)	Phenelzine
	(1192)	Tranylcypromine
	(397)	Iprindol
	(994)	Trazodone
		Nomifensin
		L-tryptophan combined with pyridoxin and ascorbic acid
	(156)	Amitriptyline combined with
	(86)	Perphenazine
	(156)	Amitriptyline combined with
	(523)	Chlordiazepoxide
	(47)	Fluphenazine dihydrochloride combined with
	(223)	Nortriptyline
	(1192)	Tranylcypromine (10 mg) combined with
	(130)	Trifluoperazine (1 mg)
Secondary:	(100)	Propericiazine

4.5. Depressive syndrome with delusions and hallucinations

Psychopathology. In contrast to schizophrenic reactions, the content of delusions and hallucinations is congruent with the depressive affect; for instance, voices accusing the patient because he feels guilty or hallucinations of being in hell or in prison are "deserved" as a punishment for his guilt. Sometimes the patient believes the police are persecuting him because of his sins. The whole content of the delusions and hallucinations is synthymic with the thought content, i.e., both are depressed. In older patients one often hears expressed ideas of poverty in respect to money, clothes, and food plus the conviction that not only the patient but also his family are dying. Such patients often express the idea that their spouse is already dead.

Pharmacological treatment. High dosages of tricyclic antidepressants, if necessary in combination with a nonsedative antipsychotic drug in lower dosages or in combination with high dosages of a minor tranquilizer such as diazepam or oxazepam. At times MAOIs alone or in combination with a tricyclic and other medications specified above are required.

Drugs indicated:

Primary:	(156)	Amitriptyline
	(245)	Trimepramine
	(227)	Opipramol
	(187)	Doxepin
	(206)	Imipramine
	(165)	Chlorimipramine (clomipramine)
	(223)	Nortriptyline
	(182)	Desipramine
	(184)	Dibenzepin
	(171)	Clofepramine (lopramine)
	(164)	Carpipramine
	(162)	Butriptyline
	(236)	Protriptyline
	(235)	Prothiaden
		Viloxazine

(1252)	Maprotiline
	Mianserine
(1259)	Tofenacine
(776)	Iproniazid
(777)	Isocarboxazide
(867)	Nialamide
(1165)	Phenelzine
(1192)	Tranylcypromine
(397)	Iprindol
(994)	Trazodone
	Nomifensin
	L-tryptophan combined with pyridoxin and ascorbic acid
(156)	Amitriptyline combined with
(86)	Perphenazine
(156)	Amitriptyline combined with
(523)	Chlordiazepoxide
(47)	Fluphenazine dihydrochloride combined with
(223)	Nortriptyline
(1192)	Tranylcypromine (10mg) combined with
(130)	Trifluoperazine
	Lithium (prophylaxis)

Secondary: (621) Haloperidol

4.6. Manic-hypomanic syndrome

Psychopathology. The syndrome is characterized by overactivity, loss of concentration, flight of ideas, disinhibition, logorrhea, elated euphoric mood, irritable behavior, inner restlessness, ecstatic feelings, and increased self-confidence, and occasionally by delusion of grandeur or sudden swings into depressive outbursts. Also characteristic are increased initiative and spontaneity, motor restlessness, increased social contact, a plethora of plans and ideas, refusal of treatment, and increased sexuality. The symptoms may show diurnal fluctuations with improvement in the evening. Sleeplessness is one of the most prominent symptoms.

Pharmacological treatment. The patient doesn't feel sick and feels no need for treatment. He feels stronger and better than ever and hence is very difficult to treat. Lithium (1000 to 2000 mg/day) is the drug of choice but usually requires four to ten days to act and therefore must be combined with sedative major tranquilizers such as clozapine, clopenthixol, levomepromazine, chlorpromazine, and haloperidol. Phenothiazines may cause dysphoria and hence other antipsychotic agents may be preferred. In rare cases it is justifiable to give haloperidol drops in tea or coffee. Sometimes it is necessary to use a depot injection of a sedative major tranquilizer: pipothiazin-palmitate, clopenthixol-decanoate. During the night a combination with barbiturates is sometimes helpful although high doses of sedative phenothiazines or clozapine are preferable. When the acute phase subsides the lithium should be continued but the other medications may be rapidly decreased.

Drugs indicated:

Primary:	(20)	Chlorpromazine
	(132)	Triflupromazine
	(69)	Levomepromazine (methotrimeprazine)
	(86)	Perphenazine
	(47)	Fluphenazine dihydrochloride
	(7)	Butaperazine
	(123)	Thiopropazate
	(130)	Trifluoperazine
	(95)	Prochlorperazine
	(4)	Acetophenazine
	(9)	Carphenazine
	(93)	Piperacetazine
	(168)	Chlorprothixene
	(173)	Clopenthixol
	(621)	Haloperidol
	(753)	Fluspirilene
	(909)	Penfluridol
	(199)	Clozapine
	(318)	Reserpine
	(1552)	Lithium (prophylaxis)
Secondary:	(608)	Benperidol

4.7. Syndrome of simultaneous manic and depressive responses

Psychopathology. Although some of the manifestations of the manic and the depressive phase are mutually exclusive, there are other symptoms which can coexist. Unless the clinician is aware of this, the picture can be very confusing. Not only can the mood swing rapidly from one extreme to the other, but a hyperactive and euphoric patient under pressure of speech may suddenly burst into tears but continue to behave in an otherwise hypomanic manner. All sorts of odd combinations are possible.

Pharmacological treatment. Combined tricyclic plus major tranquilizer medication is the most effective (e.g., perphenazine plus amitriptyline). Lithium should be started as soon as possible. Stimulant major tranquilizing agents may also be used.

Drugs indicated:

Primary:

(86)	Perphenazine
(47)	Fluphenazine dihydrochloride
(7)	Butaperazine
(123)	Thiopropazate
(130)	Trifluoperazine
(95)	Prochlorperazine
(4)	Acetophenazine
(9)	Carphenazine
(93)	Piperacetazine
(168)	Chlorprothixene
(173)	Clopenthixol
(243)	Thiothixene
(621)	Haloperidol
(199)	Clozapine
(1552)	Lithium (prophylaxis)

In combination with a major tranquilizer:

(156)	Amitriptyline
(245)	Trimipramine
(227)	Opipramol

(187) Doxepin
(206) Imipramine
(165) Chlorimipramine (clomipramine)
(223) Nortriptyline
(182) Desipramine
(184) Dibenzepin
(171) Clofepramine (lopramine)
(164) Carpipramine
(162) Butriptyline
(236) Protriptyline
(235) Prothiaden
       Viloxazine
(1252) Maprotiline (ludiomil)
       Mianserine
(1259) Tofenacine
(776) Iproniazid
(777) Isocarboxazide
(867) Nialamide
(1165) Phenelzine
(1192) Tranylcypromine
(397) Iprindol
(994) Trazodone
       Nomifensin
       L-tryptophan combined with
       pyridoxin and ascorbic acid
(156) Amitriptyline combined with
(86)   Perphenazine
(156) Amitriptyline combined with
(523) Chlordiazepoxide
(47)   Fluphenazine dihydrochloride combined
       with
(223) Nortriptyline
(1192) Tranylcypromine (10 mg) combined with
(130) Trifluoperazine

Secondary: (20)   Chlorpromazine
(132) Triflupromazine

5. NEUROTIC AND PERSONALITY DISORDER SYNDROMES

5.1. Anxiety state or syndrome

Psychopathology. The anxiety state is characterized by excessive anxiety often amounting to panic. It can manifest itself in the psychic sphere or in the somatic field with autonomic reactions. The patient often suffers from free-floating anxiety with cardiovascular symptoms (tachycardia, palpitations, feelings of faintness) and dryness of the mouth, lack of appetite, dyspepsia, fullness of the stomach, gastric pain before or after meals, nausea, and occasionally vomiting. The anxiety may be increased under certain circumstances such as crowded surroundings. The patient is agitated to varying degrees.

Anxiety states tend to be overdiagnosed; the true underlying diagnosis of depression is very often missed. Many depressive syndromes show marked symptoms of anxiety and even agitation. There is rarely depression without anxiety, so what appears to be an anxiety state must be very closely examined to determine whether it is actually an agitated depression. At the end of one to two months of treatment, if the patient diagnosed as having an anxiety state experiences no relief, one ought to reexamine the case to see whether there is not an underlying depression. Look for basic symptoms of a depressive state: symptoms worse in the morning and better in the evening, early awakening, and so on.

Pharmacological treatment. In milder cases the treatment of choice is a minor tranquilizer. One has to beware of the development of tolerance and the risk of psychological dependence. This is unlikely to occur at low doses, but there is a risk of the patient escalating the dose. Therefore after two or three months these medications should gradually be withheld if the dose is above the minimal level. One should switch to such sedative antidepressants as doxepine, and opipramol, or to sedative major tranquilizers (promazine, thioridazine, levomepromazine, clozapine, chlorprothixene). One can try a combination of perphenazine and amitriptyline or an MAOI. If the patient does not respond to antianxiety pharmacological treatment within two to three months, one has to think of depression; if this is excluded, the patient should be referred for possible psychotherapy. Chronic anxiety states of neurotic origin provide only a limited indication for medication.

Drugs indicated:

Primary:	(98)	Promazine
	(20)	Chlorpromazine
	(132)	Triflupromazine
	(69)	Levomepromazine (methotrimeprazine)
	(938)	Prothipendyl
	(168)	Chlorprothixene
	(243)	Thiothixene
	(522)	Chlorazepate
	(523)	Chlordiazepoxide
	(528)	Diazepam
	(533)	Lorazepam
	(534)	Medazepam
	(538)	Oxazepam
	(1446)	Meprobamate
	(768)	Hydroxyzine
		Hydroxyzine pamoate
	(1470)	Methylpentynol
	(1447)	Methylpentynol carbamate
	(1104)	Benzoctamine
	(704)	Chlormethazanone
	(938)	Prothipendyl
	(1361)	Methocarbamol

(1451) Tybamate
(1212) Benactyzine
(1371) Phenaglycodol
(1242) Captodiame
(1244) Diphenhydramine

Combinations (see table,§ **14**)

Secondary: (125) Thioridazine
(65) Mesoridazine
(100) Propericiazine
(173) Clopenthixol
(191) Flupenthixol
(621) Haloperidol
(199) Clozapine
(776) Iproniazid
(777) Isocarboxazide
(867) Nialamide
(1165) Phenelzine
(1192) Tranylcypromine
(1192) Tranylcypromine (10 mg) combined with
(130) Trifluoperazine (1 mg.)

5.2. Phobic and obsessive-compulsive syndrome

Psychopathology. Characteristic is a sense of subjective compulsion to follow a recurring idea or train of thought which may be nonsensical and takes the form of rumination which the patient attempts in vain to dispel; or the repetition of an activity which the patient feels compelled to carry out. There may be severe anxiety, especially when obsessive-compulsive activity is resisted or otherwise interfered with. Phobic symptoms are characterized by intense dread, often amounting to panic, in the presence of an object or a situation, e.g., dread of open or closed spaces.

Pharmacological treatment. MAOIs are probably the most effective available treatment. Alternatives are propericiazine, clozapine, minor tranquilizers, and possibly amitriptyline. Other psychotropic drugs, however, are not very effective.

Drugs indicated:

Primary:	(938)	Prothipendyl
	(156)	Amitriptyline
	(245)	Trimepramine
	(227)	Opipramol
	(187)	Doxepin
	(206)	Imipramine
	(165)	Chlorimipramine (clomipramine)
	(223)	Nortriptyline
	(182)	Desipramine
	(184)	Dibenzepin
	(171)	Clofepramine (lopramine)
	(164)	Carpipramine
	(162)	Butriptyline
	(236)	Protriptyline
	(235)	Prothiaden
		Viloxazine
	(1252)	Maprotiline
		Mianserine
	(1259)	Tofenacine
	(776)	Iproniazid
	(777)	Isocarboxazide
	(867)	Nialamide
	(1165)	Phenelzine
	(1192)	Tranylcypramine
	(397)	Iprindol
	(994)	Trazodone
		Nomifensin
		L-tryptophan combined with pyridoxin and ascorbic acid
	(156)	Amitriptyline combined with
	(86)	Perphenazine
	(156)	Amitriptyline combined with
	(523)	Chlordiazepoxide
	(47)	Fluphenazine dihydrochloride combined with

      (223)   Nortriptyline
    (1192)   Tranylcypromine (10 mg) combined with
      (130)   Trifluoperazine (1 mg)

Secondary: (20)   Chlorpromazine
      (132)   Triflupromazine
      (125)   Thioridazine
       (65)   Mesoridazine
      (191)   Flupenthixol
      (522)   Chlorazepate
      (523)   Chlordiazepoxide
      (528)   Diazepam
      (533)   Lorazepam
      (534)   Medazepam
      (538)   Oxazepam
    (1446)   Meprobamate
      (768)   Hydroxyzine
              Hydroxyzine pamoate
    (1470)   Methylpentynol
    (1447)   Methylpentynol carbamate
    (1104)   Benzoctamine
      (704)   Chlormethazanone
      (938)   Prothipendyl
    (1361)   Methocarbamol
    (1451)   Tybamate
    (1212)   Benactyzine
    (1371)   Phenaglycodol
    (1242)   Captodiame
    (1244)   Diphenhydramine

Combinations (see table, § **14**)

5.2.1. Gilles de la Tourette syndrome

Multiple tics predominantly of the face or neck connected with obsessive-compulsive actions and obscene exclamations including coprolalia. The syndrome most frequently starts between the ages of seven and eight with motor tics in the face (oral and ocular motor tics) spreading later to the shoulders and arms; these may finally be generalized to the whole body. In a later stage there are tics of phonation, i.e., the uttering or bursting out of phrases or words that frequently are obscene (coprolalia) or repetitive (echolalia). As a rule the syndrome starts before the age of sixteen. The etiology may by psychosocial or cerebral organic (the latter especially in adults after encephalitis).

Pharmacological treatment.   According to Snyder (218), blocking of dopamine receptors in the brain is one of the most effective treatments.

Drugs indicated:

> *Primary*:   (621)   Haloperidol

> *Secondary*:   none

5.2.2. Anorectic syndrome

Psychopathology.   Severe weight loss induced in anorexia nervosa by attempts at dieting for the sake of slimness but finally to avoid increase of weight and physical maturation; it is often connected with vomiting, abuse of laxatives or other drugs, chronic obstipation, and secondary amenorrhea. The syndrome is also to be found secondary to drug abuse, loss of appetite in depressive states, and denial of food in schizophrenia.

Pharmacological treatment.   The most important treatment usually is psychotherapy. But in urgent cases it may be necessary to feed the patient artificially. In these cases a tube has to be placed into the stomach together with high dosages of sedative major tranquilizers. On other occasions there appears to be underlying depression, and the antidepressant drugs, especially the MAOIs, have proved useful.

Drugs indicated:

> *Primary*:   (69)   Levomepromazine (methotrimeprazine)

> *Secondary*:   (20)   Chlorpromazine

5.3. Depressive neurotic syndrome

Psychopathology. The depression follows some acute psychic trauma or develops as a result of chronic psychological conflict. The symptomatology shows rapid changes dependent on the external situation and is often linked with symptoms of aggression or appeals to others. The symptoms tend to be worse in the evening, and the patient has difficulty falling asleep. Mixed in with symptoms of anxiety there is often hostility.

Pharmacological treatment. The patient is less likely to respond to medication than is the case with other forms of depression. If there is no improvement within two months, consider psychotherapy. MAOIs may be useful if there is dysphoria. Otherwise use tricyclic antidepressants (amitriptyline, maprotiline, nortriptyline, opipramol) or combine nortriptyline with amitriptyline, doxepine, and protriptyline. Give doxepine or a combination of amitriptyline and chlordiazepoxide.

Drugs indicated:

Primary :	(156)	Amitriptyline
	(245)	Trimepramine
	(227)	Opipramol
	(187)	Doxepin
	(206)	Imipramine
	(165)	Chlorimipramine (clomipramine)
	(223)	Nortriptyline
	(182)	Desipramine
	(184)	Dibenzepin
	(171)	Clofepramine (lopramine)
	(164)	Carpipramine
	(162)	Butriptyline
	(136)	Protriptyline
	(235)	Prothiaden
		Viloxazine
	(1252)	Maprotiline
		Mianserine
	(1259)	Tofenacine

(776)	Iproniazid
(777)	Isocarboxazide
(867)	Nialamide
(1165)	Phenelzine
(1192)	Tranylcypromine
(397)	Iprindol
(994)	Trazodone
	Nomifensin
	L-tryptophan combined with pyridoxin and ascorbic acid
(156)	Amitriptyline combined with
(86)	Perphenazine
(156)	Amitriptyline combined with
(523)	Chlordiazepoxide
(47)	Fluphenazine dihydrochloride combined with
(223)	Nortriptyline
(1192)	Tranylcypromine (10 mg) combined with
(130)	Trifluoperazine (1 mg)

Secondary:	(125)	Thioridazine
	(65)	Mesoridazine
	(191)	Flupenthixol
	(1098)	Dextroamphetamine
	(1147)	Methamphetamine
		Methylphenidate
	(931)	Piperadrol
	(1147)	Methamphetamine combined with
	(563)	Amobarbital
	(1147)	Methamphetamine combined with
		Phenobarbital-Na
	(1098)	Dextroamphetamine combined with
	(563)	Amobarbital
	(522)	Chlorazepate
	(523)	Chlordiazepoxide
	(528)	Diazepam
	(533)	Lorazepam
	(534)	Medazepam
	(538)	Oxazepam
	(1446)	Meprobamate

(768)	Hydroxyzine
	Hydroxyzine pamoate
(1470)	Methylpentynol
(1447)	Methylpentynol carbamate
(1104)	Benzoctamine
(704)	Chlormethazanone
(938)	Prothipendyl
(1361)	Methocarbamol
(1451)	Tybamate
(1212)	Benactyzine
(1371)	Phenaglycodol
(1242)	Captodiame
(1244)	Diphenhydramine
(1552)	Lithium (prophylaxis)

Combinations (see table, § 14)

5.4. Neurotic hypochondriacal syndrome

Psychopathology. Persistent anxiety is present plus a preoccupation and overconcern with physical and at times mental health. The condition tends to be chronic, with a vicious circle of reinforcement of the anxiety because of self-observation of unimportant autonomic symptoms.

Pharmacological treatment. Whatever medication is used should be started at a very low dose and built up slowly, because this type of patient tolerates side effects so very poorly. Possibly tryptophane should be tried first because it has so few side effects. Also to be considered are opipramol, doxepin, and amitriptyline. Diazepam and chlordiazepoxide may be combined in cases of anxiety attacks. Give a drug for at least four weeks, since frequent change of medication increases the patient's insecurity. Explain the side effects if they appear; inform the patient, beforehand if possible, about the most frequent side effects (dryness of mouth, disturbance of accommodation and sweating) to forestall anxiety. In cases where side effects result in the patient's discontinuing medication, low doses of MAOIs may be started, gradually increasing to a full dose as needed.

Drugs indicated:

Primary:	(168)	Chlorprothixene
	(156)	Amitriptyline
	(245)	Trimepramine
	(227)	Opipramol
	(187)	Doxepin
	(206)	Imipramine
	(165)	Chlorimipramine (clomipramine)
	(223)	Nortriptyline
	(182)	Desipramine
	(184)	Dibenzepin
	(171)	Clofepramine (lopramine)
	(164)	Carpiparmine
	(162)	Butriptyline
	(236)	Protriptyline
	(235)	Prothiaden
		Viloxazine
	(1252)	Maprotiline
		Mianserine
	(1259)	Tofenacine
	(397)	Iprindol
	(994)	Trazodone
		Nomifensin
		L-tryptophan combined with pyridoxin and ascorbic acid
	(156)	Amitriptyline combined with
	(86)	Perphenazine
	(156)	Amitriptyline combined with
	(523)	Chlordiazepoxide
	(47)	Fluphenazine dihydrochloride combined with
	(223)	Nortriptyline
	(522)	Chlorazepate
	(523)	Chlordiazepoxide
	(528)	Diazepam
	(533)	Lorazepam
	(534)	Medazepam

(538) Oxazepam
(1446) Meprobamate
(768) Hydroxyzine
       Hydroxyzine pamoate
(1470) Methylpentynol
(1447) Methylpentynol carbamate
(1104) Benzoctamine
(704) Chlormethazanone
(938) Prothipendyl
(1361) Methocarbamol
(1451) Tybamate
(1212) Benactyzine
(1371) Phenaglycodol
(1242) Captodiame
(1244) Diphenhydramine

Combinations (see table, § **14**)

Secondary: (125) Thioridazine
       (65) Mesoridazine
       (199) Clozapine
       (776) Iproniazid
       (777) Isocarboxazide
       (867) Nialamide
       (1165) Phenelzine
       (1192) Tranylcypromine
       (1192) Tranylcypromine (10 mg) combined with
       (130) Trifluoperazine (1 mg)
       (1552) Lithium (prophylaxis)

5.5. Hysterical syndrome

Psychopathology. Many other syndromes have hysterical features, but pure hysteria is a rare diagnosis made only if there is a background of an hysterical personality with affective immaturity and affective instability; there are inappropriate reactions to emotional stimuli, impulsive enthusiasms, easily provoked laughter and tears, rapid changes in mood, lack of real depth of emotions, and egocentricity. The whole external world is seen only in the light of the patient's own interests. He or she is possessive, tends to provoke passionate scenes laden with accusations, tears, protestations, and reconciliations which exhaust everyone else involved. The histrionic facet of the personality tends to dramatize and seek out the attention of others.

Pharmacological treatment.   In acute hysteric attacks use minor tranquilizers i.v., although these are without any long-term effect. Sometimes long-term treatment with neuleptil, clozapine, etc. may be useful. After excluding any underlying more serious psychotic disorder, refer the patient for psychotherapy.

Drugs indicated:

Primary:	(20)	Chlorpromazine
	(132)	Triflupromazine
	(69)	Levomepromazine (methotrimeprazine)
	(100)	Propericiazine
	(168)	Chlorprothixene
	(522)	Chlorazepate
	(523)	Chlordiazepoxide
	(528)	Diazepam
	(533)	Lorazepam
	(534)	Medazepam
	(538)	Oxazepam
	(1446)	Meprobamate
	(768)	Hydroxyzine
		Hydroxyzine pamoate
	(1470)	Methylpentynol
	(1447)	Methylpentynol carbamate
	(1104)	Benzoctamine
	(704)	Chlormethazanone
	(938)	Prothipendyl
	(1361)	Methocarbamol
	(1451)	Tybamate
	(1212)	Benactyzine

	(1371)	Phenaglycodol
	(1242)	Captodiame
	(1244)	Diphenhydramine

Combinations (see table, § **14**)

Secondary: (199) Clozapine

(156)	Amitriptyline
(245)	Trimepramine
(227)	Opipramol
(187)	Doxepin
(206)	Imipramine
(165)	Chlorimipramine (clomipramine)
(223)	Nortriptyline
(182)	Desipramine
(184)	Dibenzepin
(171)	Clofepramine (lopramine)
(164)	Carpipramine
(162)	Butriptyline
(236)	Protriptyline
(235)	Prothiaden
	Viloxazine
(1252)	Maprotiline
	Mianserine
(1259)	Tofenacine
(397)	Iprindol
(994)	Trazodone
	Nomifensin
	L-tryptophan combined with pyridoxin and ascorbic acid
(156)	Amitriptyline combined with
(86)	Perphenazine
(156)	Amitriptyline combined with
(523)	Chlordiazepoxide
(47)	Fluphenazine dihydrochloride combined with
(223)	Nortriptyline

5.5.1. Ganser's syndrome

Psychopathology. A very rare state of hysterical pseudodementia simulating a pseudostupidity, showing retarded behavior, and giving predominantly inane answers to simple questions, in which the patient (unconsciously) simulates a psychosis. This hysterical syndrome is frequently connected with the obvious aim of avoiding punishment or other unfavorable judgments. A similar syndrome is observed in children as a regressive phenomenon to earlier motor and verbal behavior.

Pharmacological treatment. The most important treatment is psychotherapy. At the beginning it can be combined with major or minor tranquilizers.

Drugs indicated:

Primary:	(20)	Chlorpromazine
	(132)	Triflupromazine
	(69)	Levomepromazine (methotrimeprazine)
	(100)	Propericiazine
	(168)	Chlorprothixene
	(522)	Chlorazepate
	(528)	Diazepam
	(533)	Lorazepam
	(534)	Medazepam
	(538)	Oxazepam
	(1446)	Meprobamate
	(768)	Hydroxyzine
		Hydroxyzine pamoate
	(1470)	Methylpentynol
	(1447)	Methylpentynol carbamate
	(1104)	Benzoctamine
	(704)	Chlormethazanone
	(938)	Prothipendyl
	(1361)	Methocarbamol
	(1451)	Tybamate
	(1212)	Benactyzine

(1371) Phenaglycodol
(1242) Captodiame
(1244) Diphenhydramine

Combinations (see table, § 14)

Secondary: (199) Clozapine
(156) Amitriptyline
(245) Trimepramine
(227) Opipramol
(187) Doxepin
(206) Imipramine
(165) Chlorimipramine (clomipramine)
(223) Nortriptyline
(182) Desipramine
(184) Dibenzepin
(171) Clofepramine (lopramine)
(164) Carpipramine
(162) Butriptyline
(236) Protriptyline
(235) Prothiaden
       Viloxazine
(1252) Maprotiline
       Mianserine
(1259) Tofenacine
(397) Iprindol
(994) Trazodone
       Nomifensin
       L-tryptophan combined with
       pyridoxin and ascorbic acid
(156) Amitriptyline combined with
(86) Perphenazine
(156) Amitriptyline combined with
(523) Chlordiazepoxide
(47) Fluphenazine dihydrochloride
       combined with
(223) Nortriptyline

5.5.2. Multiple personality

Psychopathology. The syndrome of dissociative behavior in hysteria may lead to the coexistence in a patient of behavior and personality traits of two or more different persons with or without amnesia as to the existence of the other "personalities." Very often this occurs as an understandable escape from a disagreeable situation. Medical and public attention may aggravate the manifestation.

Pharmacological treatment. Not indicated.

5.6. Neurasthenic syndrome

Psychopathology. Symptoms of irritability, weakness, rapid exhaustion, fatigue, sleep disturbances, loss of sexual potency, lack of drive and energy, functional loss of memory, headache, dizziness, autonomic symptoms of the gastrointestinal tract or cardiovascular system.

Pharmacological treatment. Mild sedative tricyclic or tetracyclic antidepressants possibly in combination with a minor tranquilizer. If this is without benefit, there are occasions when an MAOI will succeed.

Drugs indicated:

Primary:	(156)	Amitriptyline
	(245)	Trimepramine
	(227)	Opipramol
	(187)	Doxepin
	(206)	Imipramine
	(165)	Chlorimipramine (clomipramine)
	(223)	Nortriptyline
	(182)	Desipramine
	(184)	Dibenzepin
	(171)	Clofepramine (lopramine)
	(164)	Carpipramine
	(162)	Butriptyline
	(236)	Protriptyline

(235)   Prothiaden
        Viloxazine
(1252) Maprotiline
        Mianserine
(1259) Tofenacine
(397)   Iprindol
(994)   Trazodone
        Nomifensin
        L-tryptophan combined with
        pyridoxin and ascorbic acid
(156)   Amitriptyline combined with
(86)   Perphenazine
(156)   Amitriptaline combined with
(523)   Chlordiazepoxide
(47)   Fluphenazine dihydrochloride combined
        with
(223)   Nortriptyline

Secondary: (522)   Chlorazepate
              (523)   Chlordiazepoxide
              (528)   Diazepam
              (533)   Lorazepam
              (534)   Medazepam
              (538)   Oxazepam
             (1446)   Meprobamate
              (768)   Hydroxyzine
                      Hydroxyzine pamoate
             (1470)   Methylpentynol
             (1447)   Methylpentynol carbamate
             (1104)   Benzoctamine
              (704)   Chlormethazanone
              (938)   Prothipendyl
             (1361)   Methocarbamol
             (1451)   Tybamate
             (1212)   Benactyzine
             (1371)   Phenaglycodol
             (1242)   Captodiame
             (1244)   Diphenhydramine

        Combinations (see table, § **14**)

5.7. Sexual neurotic syndrome

Psychopathology. Excessive or aberrant sexual behavior usually involves biological, intrapersonal, and social factors. To some degree the culture in which the activity takes place provides the criterion as to whether or not the behavior is "neurotic" (usually a pejorative or explicatory substitute for the word *abnormal*).

Pharmacological treatment. Refer patients for psychotherapy or behavioral therapy or sex therapy. In cases of sexual hyperactivity an antiandrogen or a minor tranquilizer is useful. In cases of premature ejaculation try an MAOI in very low doses to decrease sensitivity; higher doses of MAOIs may lead to impotence. Benperidol has been recommended for hyperactivity difficult to control.

Drugs indicated:

    Primary: (100)   Propericiazine
                      (608)   Benperidol

            In combination with a major tranquilizer:

                      (156)   Amitriptyline
                      (245)   Trimepramine
                      (227)   Opipramol
                      (187)   Doxepin
                      (206)   Imipramine
                      (165)   Chlorimipramine (clomipramine)
                      (223)   Nortriptyline
                      (182)   Desipramine
                      (184)   Dibenzepin
                      (171)   Clofepramine (lopramine)
                      (164)   Carpipramine
                      (162)   Butriptyline
                      (236)   Protriptyline
                      (235)   Prothiaden
                              Viloxazine
                     (1252)   Maprotiline
                              Mianserine
                     (1259)   Tofenacine
                      (776)   Iproniazid

	(777)	Isocarboxazide
	(867)	Nialamide
	(1165)	Phenelzine
	(1192)	Tranylcypromine
	(397)	Iprindol
	(994)	Trazodone
		Nomifensin
		L-tryptophan combined with pyridoxin and ascorbic acid
	(156)	Amitriptyline combined with
	(86)	Perphenazine
	(156)	Amitriptyline combined with
	(523)	Chlordiazepoxide
	(47)	Fluphenazine dihydrochloride combined with
	(223)	Nortriptyline
	(1192)	Tranylcypromine (10 mg) combined with
	(130)	Trifluoperazine (1 mg)
Secondary:	(522)	Chlorazepate
	(523)	Chlordiazepoxide
	(528)	Diazepam
	(533)	Lorazepam
	(534)	Medazepam
	(538)	Oxazepam
	(1446)	Meprobamate
	(768)	Hydroxyzine
		Hydroxyzine pamoate
	(1470)	Methylpentynol
	(1447)	Methylpentynol carbamate
	(1104)	Benzoctamine
	(704)	Chlormethazanone
	(938)	Prothipendyl
	(1361)	Methocarbamol
	(1451)	Tybamate
	(1212)	Benactyzine
	(1371)	Phenaglycodol
	(1242)	Captodiame
	(1244)	Diphenhydramine

Combinations (see table, § 14)

6. BRAIN DISORDER SYNDROMES

The primary symptoms of the organic brain syndromes are impairment of recent and remote memory, deficit in immediate recall, disorientation, and impairment of intellectual functions (for instance, comprehension, problem solving, and learning). Further characteristics are lability of affect and poor control of drive and mood. This syndrome accounts for over 20 percent of all first admissions to mental hospitals in the United States and approximately 10 percent of the resident population. There may be about three million persons suffering from such disorders in the age group over 65. The incidence is expected to increase in the future.

6.1. Principles of treatment

The treatment of organic brain syndromes is very difficult. From a methodological point of view the effect of most of the substances being used has not been "scientifically" demonstrated, but this does not exclude successful results in single cases. Avoid as long as possible any sedative or tranquilizing agents. All of them may lower the cerebral blood supply. The application of other drugs (tranquilizers, hypnotics) requires cautiousness in dosage because patients with organic brain syndrome have a lower tolerance to drugs.

All pharmacological treatments have to be given for at least several months until an effect can be expected. Start with low dosages and increase slowly.

6.2. Pharmacotherapy

Symptomatic pharmacotherapy of mood alterations, disturbed sleep, psychotic behavior, etc., is not treated in this section (see other syndromes). Important attempts have been made to influence the cerebral supply by (a) vasodilators, (b) stimulants, (c) cardiac therapy, and (d) antidepressants.

Vasodilators (which relax the smooth muscle of the blood vessel wall) are not specific, and even if they produce a peripheral effect this does not necessarily mean that there is also a central one in the brain. Usually pharmacotherapy is effective only in mild forms of the syndrome.

6.2.1. Vasodilators

1. Papaverine (Pavabid). Side effects: drowsiness, vertigo, flushing, heachache, abdominal distress, hypotension.

2. Hydergine. 1.5 mg t.i.d.
   Side effects: nasal congestion, nausea, gastric symptoms.

3. Cinnarizin. Dose: 3×25 mg to 3×75 mg per day.

4. Xanthinol-Nicotinat (Complamin, Complamin-Retard).
   Dosage: 3×150 mg to 300 mg Complamin or 2×500 mg Complamin-Retard. Side effects: flushing.

5. Nicotinyl-Alcoholtartaric (Ronicol, Ronicol-Retard).
   Dosage: 3×0.05 to 3×0.1 Ronicol or 2×1 Ronicol-Retard.

6. Cyclospasmol. 3×200 mg to 3×400 mg.

6.2.2. Stimulants

The following drugs in theory should stimulate the mental capacity by altering the metabolism of the nerve cells.

1. Pyrithioxin (Encephabol). Dosage: 3×100 mg per day.

2. Centrophenoxin (Lucidril). Dosage: 0.5 to 1.0 mg per day.

6.2.3. Cardiac therapy

Even if there is no sign of cardiac decompensation it is very often useful to give a cardiac glycoside (such as Digoxin) without any other indication than the fact that an organic brain syndrome exists.

6.2.4. Anti-depressants

Minimal evidence or even suspicion of depression is an indication for antidepressant medications since such treatment may restore the compensatory mechanisms. Frequently depression is present although not always easily detectable. In most organic brain disorder syndromes there are compensatory mechanisms which allow the individual to function in a relatively normal fashion. When depression occurs it is the compensatory mechanisms which are knocked out. As a result, the evidence of organic defect is overwhelming and often masks the depression. Recovery from depression usually results in return of the compensatory mechanisms.

6.3. Cerebral arteriosclerotic syndrome

Psychopathology. A common trait is the instability of the symptoms; there is often rapid improvement and worsening, with transitional confusional states involving reduced memory and disorientation in time and space. Emotional lability is often present but with some insight into the condition. Frequently present are overactivity, restlessness, and reversal of sleep rhythm. The memory disturbances rapidly worsen or remit as the clinical condition waxes and wanes. Usually remote memory remains more intact than memory of recent events.

Pharmacological treatment. Consider carefully the possibility of cardiac insufficiency and abnormalities of blood pressure. If present their correction should be a primary treatment goal. Avoid sedation as much as possible because it decreases the oxygen supply to the brain. For sleeplessness prescribe chloral hydrate (side effect: flatulence) or nonbarbiturate hypnotics (methyprylon, ethchlorvynol, benzquinamid, methaqualone, nitrazepan, flurazepam). Avoid barbiturates if possible (side effects: long-action cumulative effect, development of dependency, enzyme induction, depressant effect on the cardiovascular system); if their use is unavoidable, give only low dosages.

Drugs indicated:

   Primary: none

  Secondary: (98) Promazine
              (156) Amitriptyline
              (245) Trimepramine
              (227) Opipramol
              (187) Doxepin
              (206) Imipramine
              (165) Chlorimipramine (clomipramine)
              (223) Nortriptyline
               (182) Desipramine
              (184) Dibenzepin
              (171) Clofepramine (lopramine)
              (164) Carpipramine
              (162) Butriptyline
              (236) Protriptyline
              (235) Prothiaden
                     Viloxazine
            (1252) Maprotiline
                     Mianserine
            (1259) Tofenacine
              (397) Iprindol
              (994) Trazodone
                     Nomifensin
                     L-tryptophan combined with pyridoxin and ascorbic acid
              (156) Amitriptyline combined with
               (86) Perphenazine
              (156) Amitriptyline combined with
              (523) Chlordiazepoxide
               (47) Fluphenazine dihydrochloride combined with
              (223) Nortriptyline
               (522) Chlorazepate

(523)	Chlordiazepoxide
(528)	Diazepam
(533)	Lorazepam
(534)	Medazepam
(538)	Oxazepam
(1446)	Meprobamate
(768)	Hydroxyzine
	Hydroxyzine pamoate
(1470)	Methylpentynol
(1447)	Methylpentynol carbamate
(1104)	Benzoctamine
(704)	Chlormethazanone
(938)	Prothipendyl
(1361)	Methocarbamol
(1451)	Tybamate
(1212)	Benactyzine
(1371)	Phenaglycodol
(1242)	Captodiame
(1244)	Diphenhydramine

Combinations (see table, § **14**)

6.4 Amnestic syndrome of senile dementia

Psychopathology. Severe memory disturbance is the outstanding feature together with lack of orientation in respect to time, place, and person, loss of interest, apathy, withdrawal, lack of ideas, and sometimes depression, anergy, and self-neglect. In contrast to the arteriosclerotic syndrome there are not the marked fluctuations in performance and thinking.

Pharmacological treatment. Even if the patient is senile or arteriosclerotic on the surface, there may be an underlying depression. Treatment with antidepressants may therefore be worth a trial even though the depression is not obvious. Low dosages of tricyclic antidepressants, trazodone, or MAOIs are sometimes useful. The amnestic syndrome as such takes a chronic course and cannot be influenced significantly with presently available medications. Marginal brain tissue that is functionally impaired may be restored to a more active role, which may in some cases make a difference. Antidepressants will often improve the mood even if they effect no change in the basic pathology.

Patients with organic brain syndromes (areteriosclerosis, senile dementia, etc.) are much more sensitive to drugs. Be careful with phenothiazines and minor tranquilizers, starting with lower than usual doses. Sometimes useful are vasodilators: cyclandelate (Hydergine, a mixture of dihydroergocristine, d–h–c cornine and d–h–c–kryptine), papaverine, cinnarizin, xanthinol-nicotinate (Complamin), nicotinyl-alcoholtartaric (Ronicol). Sometimes a stimulant is useful, for instance, pyritinol (Encephabol) or centrophenoxin (Lucidril). Even if there is no sign of cardiac decompensation, it is very often useful to give a cardiac glycoside without any other indication than the senile dementia brain syndrome.

Drugs indicated:

  Primary: none

  Secondary: (98)   Promazine
                 (156)   Amitriptyline
                 (245)   Trimepramine
                 (227)   Opipramol
                 (187)   Doxepin
                 (206)   Imipramine
                 (165)   Chlorimipramine (clomipramine)
                 (223)   Nortriptyline
                 (182)   Desipramine
                 (184)   Dibenzepin
                 (171)   Clofepramine (lopramine)
                 (164)   Carpipramine
                 (162)   Butriptyline
                 (236)   Protriptyline
                 (235)   Prothiaden
                         Viloxazine
                (1252)   Maprotiline
                         Mianserine
                (1259)   Tofenacine
                 (397)   Iprindol
                 (994)   Trazodone

Nomifensin
L-tryptophan combined with
pyridoxin and ascorbic acid
(156) Amitriptyline combined with
(86) Perphenazine
(156) Amitriptyline combined with
(523) Chlordiazepoxide
(47) Fluphenazine dihydrochloride combined
with
(223) Nortriptyline

6.5. Affective type of organic brain syndrome

Psychopathology. Marked loss of memory is present but the behavior is cheerful, characterized by loss of control of affect, quick changes of mood, confabulations, and hyperactivity.

Pharmacological treatment. Drugs are not primarily indicated. Give agents to increase the cerebral circulation as in arteriosclerosis. Give minor tranquilizers only if unavoidable. In cases of marked hyperactivity a sedative antipsychotic agent may be necessary.

Drugs indicated:

Primary: none

Secondary: (156) Amitriptyline
(245) Trimepramine
(227) Opipramol
(187) Doxepin
(206) Imipramine
(165) Chlorimipramine (clomipramine)
(223) Nortriptyline
(182) Desipramine
(184) Dibenzepin
(171) Clofepramine (lopramine)
(164) Carpipramine
(162) Butriptyline
(236) Protriptyline
(235) Prothiaden

           Viloxazine
(1252)   Maprotiline
           Mianserine
(1259)   Tofenacine
 (397)   Iprindol
 (994)   Trazodone
           Nomifensin
           L-tryptophan combined with
           pyridoxin and ascorbic acid
 (156)   Amitriptyline combined with
  (86)   Perphenazine
 (156)   Amitriptyline combined with
 (523)   Chlordiazepoxide
  (47)   Fluphenazine dihydrochloride combined
           with
 (223)   Nortriptyline
  (20)   Chlorpromazine
 (132)   Triflupromazine
 (125)   Thioridazine
  (65)   Mesoridazine
 (168)   Chlorprothixene
 (191)   Flupenthixol
 (522)   Chlorazepate
 (523)   Chlordiazepoxide
 (528)   Diazepam
 (533)   Lorazepam
 (534)   Medazepam
 (538)   Oxazepam
(1446)   Meprobamate
 (768)   Hydroxyzine
           Hydroxyzine pamoate
(1470)   Methylpentynol
(1447)   Methylpentynol carbamate
(1104)   Benzoctamine
 (704)   Chlormethazanone
 (938)   Prothipendyl
(1361)   Methocarbamol
(1451)   Tybamate
(1212)   Benactyzine

(1371)   Phenaglycodol
(1242)   Captodiame
(1244)   Diphenhydramine

Combinations (see table, § **14**)

6.6. Epileptic syndromes

6.6.1. Protracted seizures associated with mental changes

6.6.1.1. Petit mal syndrome

In centrencephalic epilepsy with 3/sec. spike and wave EEG complexes, a series of seizure discharges may continue for hours or days with brief intervals.

Psychopathology. A stuporlike picture with slowing of thinking, perseverating, apathy, depressive mood, disorientation, partial amnesia, and perplexity.

EEG. Prolonged generalized bilaterally synchronous and symmetrical 3/sec. spike and wave discharge usually most pronounced over frontal areas.

Pharmacological treatment. Intravenous slowly administered 2.5–10 mg diazepam or 1 G trimethadion. This may be repeated after 10 minutes. Typically there is rapid termination of EEG and clinical symptoms.

Drugs indicated:

Primary: (528)   Diazepam (intravenously)

Secondary: none

6.6.1.2. Temporal lobe seizure syndrome (psychomotor attacks)

Psychopathology. Immense variability exists between individuals, but high stability of picture for a given patient. Change in feelings of familiarity (experience of déjà vu and jamais vu) possibly followed by delusions, hallucinations, changes of body image, and mood changes (dreamy state). Frequently there are peculiar sensations in the epigastrium, as well as autonomic symptoms such as sweating or temperature changes followed by motor automatisms, speech disturbances, or head turning to one or the other side. Usually this is followed by a period of confusion (see **6.6.2.**). Sometimes the psychomotor attack may initiate a generalized convulsive seizure. Amnesia usually exists for the period of the attack.

EEG. During the attack there are bilaterally synchronous discharges at 4–6/sec., best seen in the fronto-temporal regions. In some patients, this may be combined with temporal spikes or sharp waves. Rarely there exists bilateral generalized fast activity, sometimes without EEG abnormalities in the scalp recordings. The interictal EEG shows spike and sharp wave discharges in one or both temporal regions, or no overt pathology.

Pharmacological treatment.   Hydantoin or primidone with carbamazepine (2–4 × 50 mg).

Drugs indicated:

   Primary: (163)   Carbamazepine

   Secondary: none

6.6.2. Post-ictal epileptic syndrome

6.6.2.1. After psychomotor attacks

The duration of post-ictal confusion is commonly short (1–2 minutes). If prolonged, this condition approaches psychotic behavior. Symptoms during the attacks may be characterized as "actions." The patient behaves as if he knows what he is doing, but the behavior is strange.

Psychopathology.   Slow motor activity, automatisms (monotone speech, simple movements like nodding, knocking, etc.). Patient may show very complex behavior like grooming, dressing, undressing, housecleaning, or even taking a trip. Facial expression commonly shows strong emotions such as anxiety, anger, tension, etc. Behavior is in need of reorientation. Pupils react to light. This state commonly lasts for ½–1 hour: very rarely it may continue for days. Amnesia exists for the whole period.

EEG. Slow waves practically always without epileptic discharges, commonly with asymmetries. Rarely a normal low voltage record.

Pharmacological treatment. If known epileptic under antiepileptic medication, no special treatment. If patient is without medication, hydantoin or primidone, with carbamazepine (2–4 × 50 mg) if behavior disturbances are known to occur during seizure intervals.

Drugs indicated:

   Primary: (163)   Carbamazepine

   Secondary: none

6.6.2.2. After major seizures

Psychopathology. Slow motor activity, disorientation, clouded consciousness. No psychotic symptoms.

EEG. Diffuse slow activity, usually without epileptic discharges.

Pharmacological treatment. In known epileptics with sufficient medication, no special treatment. If patient is without medication, antiepileptic medication is indicated depending on the type of epilepsy.

6.6.3. Schizophrenia-like paranoid-hallucinatory syndrome (epileptic)

6.6.3.1. Acute schizophrenia-like paranoid-hallucinatory syndrome

Psychopathology. Hallucinations, delusions, thought disorders, no disturbance of consciousness. Psychopathology develops concomitant with disappearance of seizures, and with reoccurrence of seizures the symptoms usually vanish. The syndrome is more frequently associated with psychomotor attacks than with centrencephalic seizures.

EEG. Usually normal with increased beta activity: "Forced normalisation" (Landolt[127a]) of the EEG.

Differential diagnosis. Intoxication by antiepileptic medication (especially hydantoin) with characteristic EEG: theta and delta waves, superimposed beta activity. The patient is slow and aggressive; paranoid elements are sometimes present, but usually no hallucinations. Neuropathology: nystagmus, dysarthria, diplopia.

Pharmacological treatment. Stepwise reduction of the specific antiepileptic medication within the first 10 days, if necessary complete cessation. In case the psychosis continues, keep the patient for three weeks without any antiepileptic treatment. If no improvement, treat with psychotropic drugs as one would schizophrenia. If seizures reappear, gradually reinstate antiepileptic treatment. Beware of status epilepticus.

Drugs indicated:

Primary:	(20)	Chlorpromazine
	(132)	Triflupromazine
	(86)	Perphenazine
	(47)	Fluphenazine dihydrochloride
	(7)	Butaperazine
	(123)	Thiopropazate
	(130)	Trifluoperazine
	(95)	Prochlorperazine
	(4)	Acetophenazine
	(9)	Carphenazine
	(125)	Thioridazine
	(93)	Piperacetazine
	(65)	Mesoridazine
	(100)	Propericiazine
	(173)	Clopenthixol

(191)	Flupenthixol
(243)	Thiothixene
(621)	Haloperidol

Secondary: none

6.6.3.2. Chronic paranoid syndrome (epileptic)

Psychopathology. Sometimes complete clinical similarity to schizophrenic illness. Delusions of typical schizophrenic type (mainly delusions of grandiosity), auditory hallucinations, mood changes (i.e., depression), catatonic symptoms (grimaces, stereotypes), affective contact relatively good.

EEG. Depends upon the type of seizures which the patient had before the psychosis. More often centrencephalic type (normal background rhythms with occasional generalized spike wave complexes), less often of the temporal lobe type (focal abnormalities, continuous or intermittent).

Pharmacological treatment. Antipsychotic drugs, dependent on the specific syndrome. Treat as one would treat schizophrenia.

Drugs indicated:

Primary:		
	(20)	Chlorpromazine
	(132)	Triflupromazine
	(86)	Perphenazine
	(47)	Fluphenazine dihydrochloride
	(7)	Butaperazine
	(123)	Thiopropazate
	(130)	Trifluoperazine
	(95)	Prochlorperazine
	(4)	Acetophenazine
	(9)	Carphenazine
	(125)	Thioridazine
	(93)	Piperacetazine
	(65)	Mesoridazine
	(100)	Propericiazine

(173)   Clopenthixol
(243)   Thiothixene
(621)   Haloperidol

Secondary: none

6.6.4. Character disorder syndromes of epileptic origin

Psychopathology.   Emotional instability, irritability with unpredictable reactions, explosive emotions, sudden onset of variations of mood (duration: a few hours to a few days). Character in general: slow, circumstantial, conscientious, intellectually retarded, perseverating, egocentric, and shallow affect.

Pharmacological treatment.   Carbamazapine (2–4 × 50 mg), minor tranquilizers, nonsedative antipsychotic drugs or, if necessary, antidepressants. All these psychotropic drugs combined with specific antiepileptic medication if there are seizures.

Drugs indicated:

Primary:	(522)	Chlorzepate
	(523)	Chlordizaepoxide
	(528)	Diazepam
	(533)	Lorazepam
	(534)	Medazepam
	(538)	Oxazepam
	(1446)	Meprobamate
	(768)	Hydroxyzine
		Hydoxyzine pamoate
	(1470)	Methylppentynol
	(1447)	Methylpentynol carbamate
	(1104)	Benzoetamine
	(704)	Chlormethazanone
	(938)	Prothipendyl
	(1361)	Methocarbamol
	(1451)	Tybamate
	(1212)	Benactyzine
	(1371)	Phenaglycodol

      (1242)   Captodiame
      (1244)   Diphenhydramine

      Combinations (see table, § **14**)

Secondary: none

6.7. Post-traumatic cerebral syndromes

Psychopathology. A severe cerebral trauma may induce in mild cases a cloudiness of consciousness with slow speech and confused manner, in moderate cases a loss of consciousness for seconds or minutes with intermittent short periods of confusion and later headache and drowsiness. In moderate and severe cases there is a loss of consciousness for hours, days, or weeks with a transitional post-traumatic delirious state. In some cases there are persistent post-traumatic cerebral syndromes: post-traumatic epilepsy or post-traumatic organic brain syndromes, identical in their symptomatology to amnestic syndrome of senile dementia **6.4.** or affective type of organic brain syndrome **6.5.** Focal brain damage may also induce symptomatic epilepsy. The psychiatric syndrome most frequently observed is a change in personality or *localized brain syndrome*. This is characterized by severe changes in drive and energy; by apathy, indifference, and slowness; and by lack of spontaneity. Furthermore, there may be severe changes of mood (dysphoria, depression, euphoria), frequently connected with grandiosity, aggressiveness, or antisocial behavior. Finally, there may be a marked change of a single drive (sleep, appetite, thirst, sexuality).

Pharmacological treatment. See **6.4.**, **6.5.**, and **6.6.**

Drugs indicated:

    Primary: (156)   Amitriptyline
               (245)   Trimepramine
               (227)   Opipramol
               (187)   Doxepin
               (206)   Imipramine
               (165)   Chlorimipramine (clomipramine)

(223) Nortriptyline
(182) Desipramine
(184) Dibenzepin
(171) Clofepramine (lopramine)
(164) Carpipramine
(162) Butriptyline
(236) Protriptyline
(235) Prothiaden
      Viloxazine
(1252) Maprotiline
      Mianserine
(1259) Tofenacine
(397) Iprindol
(994) Trazodone
      Nomifensin
      L-tryptophan combined with
      pyridoxin and ascorbic acid
(156) Amitriptyline combined with
(86) Perphenazine
(156) Amitriptyline combined with
(523) Chlordiazepoxide
(47) Fluphenazine dihydrochloride combined
      with
(223) Nortriptyline
(522) Chlorazepate
(523) Chlordiazepoxide
(528) Diazepam
(533) Lorazepam
(534) Medazepam
(538) Oxazepam
(1446) Meprobamate
(768) Hydroxyzine
      Hydroxyzine pamoate
(1470) Methylpentynol
(1447) Methylpentynol carbamate
(1104) Benzoctamine
(704) Chlormethazanone
(938) Prothipendyl
(1361) Methocarbamol
(1451) Tybamate

(1212) Benactyzine
(1371) Phenaglycodol
(1242) Captodiame
(1244) Diphenhydramine
 (163) Carbamazepine

Combinations (see table, § **14**)

Secondary: (98) Promazine
              (20) Chlorpromazine
             (132) Triflupromazine
             (125) Thioridazine
              (65) Mesoridazine
             (168) Chlorprothixene
             (191) Flupenthixol

6.8. Degenerative and demyelinating brain disorder syndromes

These include Huntington's chorea, multiple sclerosis, Parkinson's disease, etc. and start with localized atrophy of special structures of the brain. The mental changes correspond to a *localized brain syndrome* identical to that found in post-traumatic cerebral syndromes: change of personality, change of drive and mood, loss of control (see **6.7.**); in later stages of the atrophic process, where more extensive parts of the brain are affected, the consequences are brain disorder syndromes of the *amnestic* (**6.4.**) or *affective* types (**6.5.**).

Pharmacological treatment.   See **6.4.**, **6.5.** In Huntington's chorea the gross movements can be controlled by the application of reserpine, nonsedative phenothiazine derivatives or butyrophenones.

Drugs indicated:

Primary: (86) Perphenazine
             (47) Fluphenazine dihydrochloride
              (7) Butaperazine
            (123) Thiopropazate
            (130) Trifluoperazine
             (95) Prochlorperazine
            (621) Haloperidol

(633) Trifluperidol
(318) Reserpine
(156) Amitriptyline
(245) Trimepramine
(227) Opipramol
(187) Doxepin
(206) Imipramine
(165) Chlorimipramine (clomipramine)
(223) Nortriptyline
(182) Desipramine
(184) Dibenzepin
(171) Clofepramine (lopramine)
(164) Carpipramine
(162) Butriptyline
(236) Protriptyline
(235) Prothiaden
      Viloxazine
(1252) Maprotiline
      Mianserine
(1259) Tofenacine
(397) Iprindol
(994) Trazodone
      Nomifensin
      L-tryptophan combined with
      pyridoxin and ascorbic acid
(156) Amitriptyline combined with
(86) Perphenazine
(156) Amitriptyline combined with
(523) Chlordiazepoxide
(47) Fluphenazine dihydrochloride combined
      with
(223) Nortriptyline

Secondary: (98) Promazine
(20) Chlorpromazine
(132) Triflupromazine
(125) Thioridazine
(65) Mesoridazine
(168) Chlorprothixene
(191) Flupenthixol

7. TOXICOMANIC SYNDROMES

7.1. Drug abuse syndrome

Psychopathology. This syndrome is characterized by dependence for emotional or mental relief upon drugs not medically prescribed or prescribed for some other purpose or taken in excessive doses. The obtaining and use of the drug becomes a central theme in the patient's existence. In advanced cases the patient cannot go about his activities until the drug has taken effect. Often the craving is so great that patients will lie, steal, or commit other immoral or illegal acts to obtain a supply.

Pharmacological treatment. In principle, toxicomania cannot be treated with psychotropic drugs, but one should always look carefully for an underlying depression. Sometimes it is even useful to treat the patient presumptively as if he were depressed. Many drugs which produce toxicomania are mild or strong euphoriants or stimulants such as cocaine and amphetamines (euphoriant drugs), alcohol, minor tranquilizers and hypnotics, barbiturates (disinhibiting drugs), opium and its derivatives (formerly used as antidepressant and antianxiety drugs), and cannabis (sometimes euphoriant and often anxiolytic). Many patients may be toxicomanic because they have been using "street drugs" to seek relief from a chronic depression. Look carefully for underlying depressive symptoms and treat these with antidepressant drugs. Obviously, the abused drug should be withdrawn, and except for the disinhibiting drugs this can be done directly. Routines for withdrawal from disinhibiting drugs are described elsewhere. Lithium may possibly be of help, but its usefulness has yet to be conclusively demonstrated.

Drugs indicated:

Primary:	(156)	Amitriptyline
	(245)	Trimepramine
	(227)	Opipramol
	(187)	Doxepin
	(206)	Imipramine
	(165)	Chlorimipramine (clomipramine)
	(223)	Nortriptyline
	(182)	Desipramine
	(184)	Dibenzepin
	(171)	Clofepramine (lopramine)
	(164)	Carpipramine
	(162)	Butriptyline
	(236)	Protriptyline
	(235)	Prothiaden
		Viloxazine
	(1252)	Maprotiline
		Mianserine
	(1259)	Tofenacine
	(397)	Iprindol
	(994)	Trazodone
		Nomifensin
		L-tryptophan combined with pyridoxin and ascorbic acid
	(156)	Amitriptyline combined with
	(86)	Perphenazine
	(156)	Amitriptyline combined with
	(523)	Chlordiazepoxide
	(47)	Fluphenazine dihydrochloride combined with
	(223)	Nortriptyline
	(522)	Chlorazepate
	(523)	Chlordiazepoxide

(528) Diazepam
(533) Lorazepam
(534) Medazepam
(538) Oxazepam
(1446) Meprobamate
(768) Hydroxyzine
Hydroxyzine pamoate
(1470) Methylpentynol
(1447) Methylpentynol carbamate
(1104) Benzoctamine
(704) Chlormethazanone
(938) Prothipendyl
(1361) Methocarbamol
(1451) Tybamate
(1212) Benactyzine
(1371) Phenaglycodol
(1242) Captodiame
(1244) Diphenhydramine

Combinations (see table, § **14**)

Secondary: (20) Chlorpromazine
(132) Triflupromazine

7.2. Chronic alcoholic syndrome

Psychopathology. Unquestionably the drug most abused is alcohol.
In the United States alone there are nine million "problem drinkers."
The pattern may vary from steady, day-to-day mild excess to the
sporadic spree drinker. The mild disinhibition which is the advantage
of alcohol used socially slides over into a dependence on the drug in
order to adjust socially at all. In severe cases the patient cannot
function without alcohol, yet the alcohol impairs the functioning.

Pharmacological treatment. Give antidepressant drugs because
there is no danger of dependence, or try long-term treatment with
lithium to produce a possible effect on mood or compulsive mechanisms. Lithium may also serve as a long-term "insurance policy"
against recurrence. Minor tranquilizers and barbiturates are not

recommended, because of pharmacological properties similar to alcohol and the danger of dependence.

Drugs indicated:

Primary:	(156)	Amitriptyline
	(245)	Trimepramine
	(227)	Opipramol
	(187)	Doxepin
	(206)	Imipramine
	(165)	Chlorimipramine (clomipramine)
	(223)	Nortriptyline
	(182)	Desipramine
	(184)	Dibenzepin
	(171)	Clofepramine (lopramine)
	(164)	Carpipramine
	(162)	Butriptyline
	(236)	Protriptyline
	(235)	Prothiaden
		Viloxazine
	(1252)	Maprotiline
		Mianserine
	(1259)	Tofenacine
	(397)	Iprindol
	(994)	Trazodone
		Nomifensin
		L-tryptophan combined with pyridoxin and ascorbic acid
	(156)	Amitriptyline combined with
	(86)	Perphenazine
	(156)	Amitriptyline combined with
	(523)	Chlordiazepoxide
	(47)	Fluphenazine dihydrochloride combined with
	(223)	Nortriptyline
Secondary:	(522)	Chlorazepate
	(523)	Chlordiazepoxide
	(528)	Diazepam

   (533) Lorazepam
   (534) Medazepam
   (538) Oxazepam
 (1446) Meprobamate
  (768) Hydroxyzine
          Hydroxyzine pamoate
 (1470) Methylpentynol
 (1447) Methylpentynol carbamate
 (1104) Benzoctamine
  (704) Chlormethazanone
  (938) Prothipendyl
 (1361) Methocarbamol
 (1451) Tybamate
 (1212) Benactyzine
 (1371) Phenaglycodol
 (1242) Captodiame
 (1244) Diphenhydramine

Combinations (see table, § **14**)

7.3. Alcohol-induced delirium syndrome

Psychopathology Motor restlessness, coarse tremor, anxiety, sometimes hallucinations (especially visual ones of small crawling objects), micropsia, and sometimes disorientation in time and space.

Pharmacological treatment. Watch the cardiovascular system and especially blood pressure. Protect the patient from infection. Give anticonvulsant such as chlormethiazol 2.0–8.0 g (hypnotic, antiepileptic, antidelirious) or diazepam 20 mg i.v.

Drugs indicated:

  Primary: (522) Chlorazepate
             (523) Chlordiazepoxide
             (528) Diazepam
             (533) Lorazepam
             (534) Medazepam
             (538) Oxazepam

(1446)   Meprobamate
(768)   Hydroxyzine
Hydroxyzine pamoate
(1470)   Methylpentynol
(1447)   Methylpentynol carbamate
(1104)   Benzoctamine
(704)   Chlormethazanone
(938)   Prothipendyl
(1361)   Methocarbamol
(1451)   Tybamate
(1212)   Benactyzine
(1371)   Phenaglycodol
(1242)   Captodiame
(1244)   Diphenhydramine

Combinations (see table, § 14)

Secondary: (98)   Promazine
(20)   Chlorpromazine
(132)   Triflupromazine

7.4. Paranoid and hallucinatory syndromes secondary to toxicomania

Psychopathology.   Chronic hallucinosis (usually voices) or ideas of persecution as a consequence of chronic alcohol consumption or amphetamine or cannabis dependence.

Pharmacological treatment.   Same as for paranoid schizophrenic syndromes.

Drugs indicated:

Primary: (20)   Chlorpromazine
(132)   Triflupromazine
(86)   Perphenazine
(47)   Fluphenazine dihydrochloride
(7)   Butaperazine
(123)   Thiopropazate
(130)   Trifluoperazine

     (95)   Prochlorperazine
      (4)   Acetophenazine
      (9)   Carphenazine
   (125)   Thioridazine
    (93)   Piperacetazine
    (65)   Mesoridazine
   (100)   Propericiazine
   (173)   Clopenthixol
   (191)   Flupenthixol
   (621)   Haloperidol
   (199)   Clozapine

Secondary: none

7.5. Withdrawal syndromes

Psychopathology. Tremor, anxiety, restlessness, autonomic symptoms; in severe cases, delirious states with visual and auditory hallucinations, sometimes epileptic seizures.

Pharmacological treatment. Withdraw the offending drug slowly, especially in cases of dependence on hypnotics or minor tranquilizers, in order to avoid epileptic attacks and delirious states. In some cases, small doses of minor tranquilizers are helpful but only rarely are they really necessary. Underlying depression should be looked for and treated.

Drugs indicated:

Primary: (20)   Chlorpromazine
           (132)   Triflupromazine
            (69)   Levomepromazine (methotrimepramine)
          (522)   Chlorazepate
          (523)   Chlordiazepoxide
          (528)   Diazepam
          (533)   Lorazepam
          (534)   Medazepam
          (538)   Oxazepam
        (1446)   Meprobamate

(768)	Hydroxyzine
	Hydroxyzine pamoate
(1470)	Methylpentynol
(1447)	Methylpentynol carbamate
(1104)	Benzoctamine
(704)	Chlormethazanone
(938)	Prothipendyl
(1361)	Methocarbamol
(1451)	Tybamate
(1212)	Benactyzine
(1371)	Phenaglycodol
(1242)	Captodiame
(1244)	Diphenhydramine

Combinations (see table, § **14**)

Secondary:	(86)	Perphenazine
	(47)	Fluphenazine dihydrochloride
	(7)	Butaperazine
	(123)	Thiopropazate
	(130)	Trifluoperazine
	(95)	Prochlorperazine
	(4)	Acetophenazine
	(9)	Carphenazine
	(93)	Piperacetazine

8. PSYCHIATRIC SYNDROMES OF CHILDHOOD

8.1. Hyperkinetic syndrome (MBD, minimal brain dysfunction)

Psychopathology   The syndrome is characterized by motor restlessness, short attention span, poor impulse control, learning difficulties, and emotional lability.

Pharmacological treatment.   Use stimulants, d-amphetamine, methylphenidate, caffeine, or tricyclic antidepressants.

Drugs indicated:

Primary:	(1098)	Dextroamphetamine
	(1147)	Methamphetamine
		Methylphenidate
	(931)	Piperadrol
	(1147)	Methamphetamine combined with
	(563)	Amobarbital
	(1147)	Methamphetamine combined with
		Phenobarbital–Na
	(1098)	Dextroamphetamine combined with
	(563)	Amobarbital

Secondary: (20)   Chlorpromazine
          (132) Triflupromazine
          (156) Amitriptyline
          (245) Trimepramine
          (227) Opipramol
          (187) Doxepin
          (206) Imipramine
          (165) Chlorimipramine (clomipramine)
          (223) Nortriptyline
          (182) Desipramine
          (184) Dibenzepin
          (171) Clofepramine (lopramine)
          (164) Carpipramine
          (162) Butriptyline
          (236) Protriptyline
          (235) Prothiaden
                 Viloxazine
         (1252) Maprotiline
                 Mianserine
         (1259) Tofenacine
          (397) Iprindol
          (994) Trazodone
                 Nomifensin
                 L-triptophan combined with
                 pyridoxin and ascorbic acid
          (156) Amitriptyline combined with
           (86) Perphenazine
          (156) Amitriptyline combined with
          (523) Chlordiazepoxide
           (47) Fluphenazine dihydrochloride combined
                 with
          (233) Nortriptyline
          (522) Chlorazepate
          (523) Chlordiazepoxide
          (528) Diazepam
          (533) Lorazepam
          (534) Medazepam
          (538) Oxazepam
         (1446) Meprobamate

(768)   Hydroxyzine
          Hydroxyzine pamoate
(1470) Methylpentynol
(1447) Methylpentynol carbamate
(1104) Benzoctamine
(704)   Chlormethazanone
(938)   Prothipendyl
(1361) Methocarbamol
(1451) Tybamate
(1212) Benactyzine
(1371) Phenaglycodol
(1242) Captodiame
(1244) Diephenhydramine

Combinations (see table, § **14**)

8.2. Enuresis nocturna syndrome

Psychopathology. Persistent bed wetting, whether physiologically or psychologically based, can be a difficult and embarrassing problem.

Pharmacological treatment. Very useful results can be obtained by treatment with tricyclic antidepressants (20–40 mg of imipramine or amitriptyline) or other antidepressants.

Drugs indicated:

Primary: (156) Amitriptyline
            (245) Trimepramine
            (227) Opipramol
            (187) Doxepin
            (206) Imipramine
            (165) Chlorimipramine (clomipramine)
            (223) Nortriptyline
            (182) Desipramine
            (184) Dibenzepin
            (171) Clofepramine (lopramine)
            (164) Carpipramine

(162) Butriptyline
(236) Protriptyline
(235) Prothiaden
       Viloxazine
(1252) Maprotiline
       Mianserine
(1259) Tofenacine
(397) Iprindol
(994) Trazodone
       Nomifensin
       L-tryptophan combined with
       pyridoxin and ascorbic acid
(156) Amitriptyline combined with
(86)   Perphenazine
(156) Amitriptyline combined with
(523) Chlordiazepoxide
(47)   Fluphenazine dihydrochloride combined
       with
(223) Nortriptyline

Secondary: none

8.3. Unmotivated retarded child syndrome

Psychopathology. Lack of motivation as part of the original pathology in the retarded child is often exaggerated by lack of social reinforcement. In addition to medications a program of rehabilitation is absolutely essential.

Pharmacological treatment. Look for depression and if present treat with tricyclic antidepressants.

Drugs indicated:

  Primary: (243) Thiothixene
              (633) Trifluperidol
              (156) Amitriptyline
              (245) Trimepramine
              (227) Opipramol
              (187) Doxepin

(206)	Imipramine
(165)	Chlorimipramine (clomipramine)
(223)	Nortriptyline
(182)	Desipramine
(184)	Dibenzepin
(171)	Clofepramine (lopramine)
(164)	Carpipramine
(162)	Butriptyline
(236)	Protriptyline
(235)	Prothiaden
	Viloxazine
(1252)	Maprotiline
	Mianserine
(1259)	Tofenacine
(397)	Iprindol
(994)	Trazodone
	Nomifensin
	L-tryptophan combined with pyridoxin and ascorbic acid
(156)	Amitriptyline combined with
(86)	Perphenazine
(156)	Amitriptyline combined with
(523)	Chlordiazepoxide
(47)	Fluphenazine dihydrochloride combined with
(223)	Nortriptyline

Secondary: (163) Carbamazepine

8.4. Syndrome of periodic episodes of disturbed behavior

Psychopathology. There are a variety of disturbances in children which occur periodically or episodically. These range from behavioral outbursts and irritability to apparently psychotic reactions.

Pharmacological treatment. If psychotherapy, behavior therapy, and other methods are unsuccessful, try long-term treatment with lithium since for unknown reasons lithium seems to "level out" these peaks and valleys.

Drugs indicated:

Primary:	(1552)	Lithium
Secondary:	(20)	Chlorpromazine
	(132)	Triflupromazine
	(522)	Chlorazepate
	(523)	Chlordiazepoxide
	(528)	Diazepam
	(533)	Lorazepam
	(534)	Medazepam
	(538)	Oxazepam
	(1446)	Meprobamate
	(768)	Hydroxyzine
		Hydroxyzine pamoate
	(1470)	Methylpentynol
	(1447)	Methylpentynol carbamate
	(1104)	Benzoctamine
	(704)	Chlormethazanone
	(938)	Prothipendyl
	(1361)	Methocarbamol
	(1451)	Tybamate
	(1212)	Benactyzine
	(1371)	Phenaglycodol
	(1242)	Captodiame
	(1244)	Diphenhydramine
	(163)	Carbamazepine

Combinations (see table, § **14**)

8.5. Autistic child syndrome

Psychopathology.   Syndrome of a different etiological origin not related to schizophrenia. In early infantile autism (112a) manifestations occur during the first months of life: failure of attachment to the mother, little or no apparent awareness of human contact, retarded speech development, and poor prognosis. Autistic personality (13a) is characterized by clumsy motor ability, usually good intelligence, egocentricity, lack of emotional contact, and highly specialized interests.

Pharmacological treatment. More important than drugs are education and psychotherapy. Drugs should be used only to treat symptoms, such as aggressiveness, mood disturbances, or loss of contact. Depending on the target syndrome, use sedative antipsychotic drugs, nonsedative antipsychotic drugs, minor tranquilizers, and antidepressants.

Drugs indicated:

Primary: none

Secondary: (86)   Perphenazine
                  (47)   Fluphenazine dihydrochloride
                  (7)   Butaperazine
                  (123) Thiopropazate
                  (130) Trifluoperazine
                  (95)   Prochlorperazine
                  (4)   Acetophenazine
                  (9)   Carphenazine
                  (93)   Piperacetazine
                  (100) Propericiazine
                  (191) Flupenthixol
                  (243) Thiothixene
                  (621) Haloperidol
                  (633) Trifluperidol
                  (925) Pimozide
                  (20)   Chlorpromazine
                  (132) Triflupromazine
                  (125) Thioridazine
                  (65)   Mesoridazine
                  (168) Chlorprothixene
                  (776) Iproniazid
                  (777) Isocarboxazide
                  (867) Nialamide
                  (1165) Phenelzine
                  (1192) Tranylcypromine
                  (1192) Tranylcypromine (10 mg) combined with
                  (130) Trifluoperazine (1 mg)

8.6. Infantile juvenile schizophrenic syndromes

Psychopathology. Before puberty such syndromes are very rare. Hebephrenic and catatonic syndromes predominate, mixed with such behavior disturbances as enuresis, encopresis, emotional outbursts, and withdrawal. Incoherence of thinking and speaking, affective incongruity, and sometimes hallucinations also occur. A classical paranoid syndrome occurs only rarely.

Pharmacological treatment. In principle, the same drugs as for adults. The drug treatment must be integrated in a whole therapeutic program (social, educative, psychotherapeutic). The dosage has to be adapted to age and weight. A rough formula is the following: 4 × age in years + 20 = percentage of the adult dose. For instance, the child is 7 years old: (4 × 7) + 20 = 48% of the adult dose. Limit the administration of the drug as much as possible, inform the parents and educators carefully, supervise the child in respect to side effects, and limit the time of administration. Choose the drug according to the predominating syndrome as in adults.

Drugs indicated:

Primary:	(86)	Perphenazine
	(47)	Fluphenazine dihydrochloride
	(7)	Butaperazine
	(123)	Thiopropazate
	(130)	Trifluoperazine
	(95)	Prochlorperazine
	(4)	Acetophenazine
	(9)	Carphenazine
	(93)	Piperacetazine
	(100)	Propericiazine
	(173)	Clopenthixol
	(191)	Flupenthixol
	(621)	Haloperidol
	(925)	Pimozide
	(199)	Clozapine

Secondary: (20)   Chlorpromazine
(132)   Triflupromazine
(125)   Thioridazine
(65)   Mesoridazine
(168)   Chlorprothixene

9. OLIGOPHRENIC SYNDROME

Psychopathology. Lack of mental comprehension with subsequent paucity of emotional expression because of deprivation of understanding. Emotional responses are otherwise normal, as is memory. Symptoms are dependent upon degree of oligophrenia.

Pharmacological treatment. Control behavioral disturbances symptomatically with sedating antipsychotic drugs such as thioridazine, levomepromazine, clozapine, or neuleptil.

Drugs indicated:

Primary:		none
Secondary:	(100)	Propericiazine
	(168)	Chlorprothixene
	(621)	Haloperidol
	(199)	Clozapine
	(522)	Chlorazepate
	(523)	Chlordiazepoxide
	(528)	Diazepam
	(533)	Lorazepam
	(534)	Medazepam
	(538)	Oxazepam
	(1446)	Meprobamate
	(768)	Hydroxyzine
		Hydroxyzine pamoate

(1470) Methylpentynol
(1447) Methylpentynol carbamate
(1104) Benzoctamine
(704) Chlormethazanone
(938) Prothipendyl
(1361) Methocarbamol
(1451) Tybamate
(1212) Benactyzine
(1371) Phenaglycodol
(1242) Captodiame
(1244) Diphenhydramine
(125) Thioridazine
(65) Mesoridazine

Combinations (see table, § 14)

10. ENDOCRINE PSYCHOSYNDROME

Included here are hyperthyroid "struma," hyperthyroid syndrome, Addison's syndrome, premenstrual syndrome, postmenopausal syndrome, etc. The endocrine psychosyndrome, described by M. Bleuler (36), does not designate a psychosis but a personality change. Such a change is similar to a focal brain disease, particularly of the brain stem and frontal lobes. The endocrine psychosyndrome is characterized by marked change of such biological drives as the urge to rest and relax or to be active; the urge to protect oneself against heat and cold; somatic sexuality or suppression of sexuality; hunger and satiation or thirst and refusal of liquids; and a primitive drive to mother and nurse others. There is also a marked change of drive (for instance, apathy) and of moods: apathetic, unstable, irritable, depressed, anxious, dysphoric. The changes in impulsiveness, arousability, drives and moods, may be lasting or, what is more characteristic, can start quite suddenly and then disappear without detectable reasons in the same abrupt way.

Pharmacological treatment. The primary treatment of course is hormonal. Psychopharmaceuticals can only be applied to stabilize mood or to activate drive according to the predominant syndrome (for instance, the depression syndromes, hypomanic syndrome). Lithium has been claimed to be useful at times for the prevention of mood changes due to endocrine disturbances, e.g., premenstrual syndromes.

Drugs indicated:

    Primary: none

    Secondary: (1552)   Lithium (Prophylaxis)

11. TREATMENT SUMMARIES

Obviously the authors have not tried every psychotropic drug for every syndrome. Equally obvious is the fact that even the entirety of the world literature on the subject does not contain such details, a problem compounded by the fact that patients ordinarily are not grouped according to syndrome. What we have therefore done is to have indicated *classes* of drugs we have found effective or which have been reported so in the literature. When in our own experience we have found one drug in a class particularly useful we have said so; this should not, however, be understood to exclude the possibility that other members of the group might be equally useful, or possibly even more so. In addition, the clinician will encounter patients who fail to respond to a drug which works in most cases but who do well on a different member of the same group.

As work in this field progresses, we hope to find studies being carried out showing relative efficacy, so that in some future edition we will be able to specify more precisely the recommended order of clinical use of particular preparations. We have therefore listed the class of drug to be used and have enclosed in parentheses any comments we mights have on specific preparations. Absence of comment most certainly does not entail absence of recommendation of the drug being tried.

2. Schizophrenic syndromes

Treatment summary

2.1. Passive paranoid schizophrenic syndrome

1. Nonsedative major tranquilizer

2.2. Florid paranoid agitated syndrome

1. Sedative major tranquilizer or
2. Levomepromazine plus nonsedative major tranquilizer

2.3. Systematic paranoid agitated syndrome

1. Sedative major tranquilizer (under guise of an hypnotic if necessary) or
2. Nonsedative, nonstimulating major tranquilizer

2.4. Catatonic schizophrenic syndrome

1. *If* withdrawn, strong nonseative major tranquilizer alone or in combination with a tricyclic or an MAOI or
2. *If* agitated or in danger of acting out, use sedative major tranquilizer (e.g., clozapine) or
3. *If* no response in severe cases use ECT

2.5. Simple schizophrenic syndrome

1. Stimulant major tranquilizing agent (e.g., thiothixene, carpipramine)

2.6. Hebephrenic schizophrenic syndrome

1. Sedative major tranquilizer

2.7. Schizophrenic withdrawal syndrome

1. Long-term stimulating major tranquilizer or
2. Combination of nonsedative major tranquilizer with tricyclic or MAOI

3. Schizoaffective syndromes

Treatment summary

3.1. Manic-schizophrenic syndrome

1. Sedative antipsychotic plus
2. lithium

3.2. Depressive-schizophrenic syndrome

1. Stimulant major tranquilizer or
2. Major tranquilizer with tricyclic antidepressant with lithium

4. Affective syndromes	**Treatment summary**
4.1. Retarded depressive syndrome	1. Tryptophan or 2. Stimulant antidepressants or 3. Combined MAOI and tricyclic or 4. Combined MAOI and tryptophan or 5. Combined tricyclic and triptophan or 6. Combined tricyyclic, MAOI, and tryptophan or 7. Unilateral ECT
4.2. Agitated depressive syndrome	1. Minor tranquilizer plus sedative antidepressant or 2. Levomepromazine or 3. Combined antidepressant and phenothiazine or other major tranquilizer
4.3. Affective hypochondriacal syndrome	1. Tryptophan or 2. Mild sedative tricyclic antidepressant or 3. Antidepressant plus minor tranquilizer
4.4. Depressed obsessive-compulsive syndrome	1. Treat as retarded or agitated depression or 2. MAOI or 3. Combined antidepressants with low doses of major tranquilizers
4.5. Depressive syndromes with delusions and hallucinations	1. High doses of tricyclics or 2. Addition of low doses of nonsedative major tranquilizers or 3. Addition of high doses of minor tranquilizers for short periods or 4. Addition of MAOIs alone or in combination with above
4.6. Manic-hypomanic syndrome	1. Sedative major tranquilizer plus 2. Lithium
4.7. Syndrome of simultaneous manic and depressive responses	1. Lithium 2. Combined tricyclic plus major tranquilizer or 3. Stimulant major tranquilizer

5. Neurotic and personality disorder syndromes

Treatment summary

5.1. Anxiety state or syndrome

1. Minor tranquilizer for up to two to three months unless very low dose or
2. Sedative antidepressants or
3. Sedative major tranquilizers in low dose or
4. Low doses of major tranquilizers plus antidepressants
5. Psychotherapy

5.2. Phobic and obsessive-compulsive syndrome

1. MAOIs or
2. Clozapine, propericiazine or
3. Tricyclic antidepressants or
4. Minor tranquilizers

5.3. Depressive neurotic syndrome

1. MAOIs
2. Tricyclics
3. Combined tricyyclic and major tranquilizer

5.4. Neurotic hypochondriacal syndrome

1. Tryptophan and/or
2. Tricyclic antidepressant
3. Addition of minor tranquilizers as needed

5.5. Hysterical syndrome

1. Minor tranquilizer during acute attacks
2. Clozapine, neuleptil and related drugs
3. Psychotherapy

5.6. Neurasthenic syndrome

1. Mild sedative tricyclic or tetracyclic antidepressants or
2. MAOIs
3. Combined with minor tranquilizers as needed

5.7. Sexual neurotic syndrome

1. Antiandrogens and if needed
2. Minor tranquilizers
3. Benperidol
4. MAOI for premature ejaculation

6. Brain Disorder Syndromes

Treatment summary

6.3. Cerebral arteriosclerotic syndrome

1. Vasodilators
2. Stimulants
3. Cardiac glycoside
4. Hypnotics (if necessary), preferably nonbarbiturate

	5. Antidepressants
	6. Minor tranquilizers
6.4. Amnetic syndrome of senile dementia	1. Antidepressants 2. Vasodilators 3. Stimulants 4. Cardiac glycoside 5. Minor tranquilizers
6.5. Affective type of organic brain syndrome	1. Vasocilators 2. If necessary, minor tranquilizers or sedative major tranquilizers
6.6. Epileptic syndromes	(In addition to specific antiepileptic drugs)
6.6.1. Protracted seizures (with mental changes)	
6.6.1.1. Petit mal	1. Diazepam i.v.
6.6.1.2. Temporal lobe seizures (psychomotor)	1. Primidone or hydantoin with carbamazepine
6.6.2. Post-ictal syndrome	
6.6.2.1. After psychomotor attacks	1. Primidone or hydantoin with carbamazepin
6.6.2.2. After major seizures	1. No specific medication indicated 2. Make certain antiepileptic drug sufficient
6.6.3. Schizophrenic-like paranoid-hallucinatory epileptic	1. Usually due to antiepileptic drug. Try gradual withdrawal 2. Major tranquilizers if necessary
6.6.3.1. Acute type	
6.6.3.2. Chronic paranoid epileptic syndrome	1. Treat as if schizophrenic
6.6.4. Character disorder syndromes	1. Carbamazepine 2. Minor tranquilizers 3. Nonsedative major tranquilizers 4. Antidepressants (if indicated)
6.7. Post-traumatic syndromes	As in 6.4., 6.5., and 6.6.
6.8. Degenerative and demyelinating brain disorder syndromes	1. See 6.4., and 6.5. 2. In Huntington's chorea use reserpine, nonsedative phenothiazines or butyrophenones

7. Toxicomanic syndrome

Treatment summary

7.1. Drug abuse syndrome

1. Treat underlying depression when it exists or is presumed to exist
2. Rarely a minor tranquilizer if indicated
3. Possibly lithium

7.2. Chronic alcoholic syndrome

1. Treat underlying depression when it exists or is presumed to exist
2. Rarely a minor tranquilizer if indicated
3. Possibly lithium

7.3. Alcohol-induced delirium syndrome

1. Anticonvulsant
2. Diazepam

7.4. Paranoid and hallucinatory syndromes secondary to toxicomania

1. Nonsedative major tranquilizer

7.5. Withdrawal syndromes

1. Anticonvulsants
2. Rarely the minor tranquilizers
3. Medication for underlying depression if it exists

8. Psychiatric syndromes of childhood

Treatment summary

8.1. Hyperkinetic syndrome (MBD, minimal brain dysfunction)

1. Stimulants and/or
2. Tricyclic antidepressants

8.2. Enuresis nocturna syndrome

1. Tricyclic antidepressants

8.3. Unmotivated retarded child syndrome

1. Tricyclic antidepressants

8.4. Syndrome of periodic episodes of disturbed behavior

1. Lithium

9. Oligophrenic Syndrome

Treatment summary

Control behavior symptomatically with major tranquilizers

10. Endocrine psychosyndromes

Treatment summary

Basic treatment is always the specific hormone indicated. Other medications must be used symptomatically

Part III. The Psycho-pharmaceuticals

12. ANTIPSYCHOTIC AGENTS

12.1. Effects and side effects

The major tranquilizers consist chemically of different structures (phenothiazines and related compounds, butyrophenones, Rauwolfia alkaloids, etc.). They all have in common a more or less marked antipsychotic activity on productive schizophrenic symptoms (hallucinations, delusions, thought disorders). In low dosages they may have tranquilizing properties similar to those of the minor tranquilizers (sedation of anxiety and tension). They differ mainly in respect to sedation and extrapyramidal or autonomic activity. They can be classified as nonsedative or sedative major tranquilizers. Within the phenothiazines, those with aliphatic side chains are more sedative than those with piperazine side chains. The former induce marked autonomic side effects more often and marked extrapyramidal side effects less often. The latter induce marked autonomic side effects less often, marked extrapyramidal effects more often. The butyrophenones are in general closer to this second group of phenothiazines.

In this part we will give only very short summaries for each compound (action, dosage, indication, contraindication) and have restricted ourselves to drugs currently on the market in the U.K., U.S., or Canada. A few additional compounds have been mentioned because the authors expect or hope that these drugs will be introduced in the near future.

It is not possible to enumerate all the observable side effects separately for each drug. These depend, of course, on the sensitivity of the patient, on dosage and duration of treatment, combination with other drugs, and so on. We will therefore enumerate only the most frequent and prominent side effects (for greater detail see Part IV):

Oversedation
Decrease in blood pressure
Tachycardia
Brachycardia
Sialarrhea
Dryness of mucosa
Disturbance of accomodation
Perspiration
Hypo- or hyperthermia
Increase of body weight
Jaundice
Leukopenia, agranulocytosis
Galactorhea, gynecomastia, amenorrhea
Loss of libido or potency
Tremor
Parkinsonian syndrome
Acute dystonia
Akathisia
Persistent dyskinesia
Epileptic seizures
Depression, apathy
Delirious states

12.2. Phenothiazines

12.2.1. Aminoalkyl-phenothiazines

PROMAZINE (98)*

Action. Quick sedative effect, especially useful for urgent sedation of psychotic agitation, mild antipsychotic effect (weaker than chlorpromazine), good tolerance.

*For trade names of drugs see tables 12., 13., 14., 15., and 16.3.

Indications. Agitation (psychotic, oligophrenic, and senile syndromes), in acute cases 100 mg intravenously. It can also be used for sedation in alcoholism and for potentiation of analgesics.

Syndromes for which indicated

Primary
(oral)

    5.1. Anxiety state or syndrome and elsewhere, where a mild sedative is indicated and there is danger of developing dependence on minor tranquilizers. Also of use for patients who overreact to ordinary phenothiazines.

(parenteral)

    2.2. Florid paranoid agitated syndrome

    5.1. Anxiety state or syndrome and other syndromes with agitation and motor excitement.

Secondary
(oral and/or parenteral)

    2.4. Catatonic schizophrenic syndrome

    6.3. Cerebral arteriosclerotic syndrome

    6.4. Amnestic syndrome of senile dementia

    6.7. Post-traumatic cerebral syndromes

    6.8. Degenerative and demyelinating brain disorder syndromes

    7.3. Alcohol induced delerium syndrome

Contraindications. Coronary disease, comatose states, sensitivity to phenothiazines.

Dosage. Outpatient: 25–600 mg; inpatient: 150–1000 mg.

CHLORPROMAZINE (20)

First neuroleptic drug, introduced into psychiatry in 1952 by Delay and Deniker (53) after the first administration as part of a "lytic cocktail" by Laborit (126) to potentiate anesthesia and by Hamon (87) and coworkers for the treatment of manic syndromes.

Action.   Sedative, antipsychotic, antiemetic.

Indications.   Chlorpromazine has been the most widely applied major tranquilizer, especially useful when strong sedation is needed. In the last few years it has partly been replaced by less sedative and stronger antipsychotic agents. This is especially true for long-term treatment. It is still very useful for the treatment of most schizophrenic and manic syndromes. The antipsychotic action is medium, the tolerance comparatively good (less marked extrapyramidal side effects than piperazine-phenothiazines). The effect has been clearly established in many double-blind studies against placebos, both in adults and in children. Newer major tranquilizers on the market have usually been compared in controlled studies to chlorpromazine, and most of them do not show any significant differences. Chlorpromazine has been combined with most of the other psychotropic drugs (minor tranquilizers, tricyclic antidepressants, MAOIs) and also with less sedative major tranquilizers. It has also been combined with ECT.

Syndromes for which indicated

Primary
(oral and parenteral)
    2.2. Florid paranoid agitated syndrome
    2.4. Catatonic schizophrenic syndrome
    3.1. Manic-schizophrenic syndrome
    4.2. Agitated depressive syndrome
    4.6. Manic-hypomanic syndrome
    5.1. Anxiety state or syndrome
    5.5. Hysterical syndrome
  5.5.1. Ganser's syndrome
6.6.3.1. Acute schizophrenia-like paranoid-hallucinatory syndrome
6.6.3.2. Chronic paranoid syndrome (epileptic)
    7.4. Paranoid and hallucinatory syndromes secondary to toxicomania
    7.5. Withdrawal syndromes

Secondary

2.3. Systematic paranoid syndrome

2.6. Hebephrenic schizophrenic syndrome

4.3. Affective hypochondriacal syndrome

4.7. Syndrome of simultaneous manic and depressive responses

Of secondary use in any syndrome if agitation or motor excitement becomes severe.

5.2. Phobic and obsessive-compulsive syndromes

5.2.2. Anoretic syndrome

6.5. Affective type of organic brain syndrome

6.6.3.1. Acute schizophrenia-like paranoid-hallucinatory syndrome

6.6.3.2. Chronic paranoid syndrome (epileptic)

6.7. Post-traumatic cerebral syndromes

6.8. Degenerative and demyelinating brain disorder syndromes

7.1. Drug abuse syndrome

7.3. Alcohol induced delirium syndrome

8.1. Hyperkinetic syndrome (MBD, minimal brain dysfunction

8.4. Syndrome of periodic episodes of disturbed behavior

8.5. Autistic child syndrome

8.6. Infantile juvenile schizophrenic syndromes

Dosage. Outpatient: 50–1000 mg; inpatient: 200–2000 mg. It has been shown that very high dosages of 2000 mg are more effective than 300 mg per day (171, 176). The intramuscular application induces infiltrations and frequently raises temperature and E.S.R. The drug can be given effectively once instead of three times daily (105).

TRIFLUPROMAZINE (132)

Action. Antipsychotic, similar to chlorpromazine and probably no difference in effectiveness from triflupromazine, chlorpromazine, perphenazine, and prochlorperazine (2).

Indications.   Acute and chronic schizophrenic syndromes in need of antipsychotic treatment and moderate sedation.

Syndromes for which indicated

Primary
(oral and parenteral)
   2.2. Florid paranoid agitated syndrome
   2.4. Catatonic schizophrenic syndrome
   3.1. Manic-schizophrenic syndrome
   4.2. Agitated depressive syndrome
   4.6. Manic-hypomanic syndrome
   5.1. Anxiety state or syndrome
   5.5. Hysterical syndrome
  5.5.1. Ganser's syndrome
6.6.3.1. Acute schizophrenia-like paranoid-hallucinatory syndrome
6.6.3.2. Chronic paranoid syndrome (epileptic)
   7.4. Paranoid and hallucinatory syndromes secondary to toxicomania
   7.5. Withdrawal syndromes

Secondary
   2.3. Systematic paranoid syndrome
   2.6. Hebephrenic schizophrenic syndrome
   4.3. Affective hypochondriacal syndrome

     Also of secondary use in any of the syndromes if agitation or motor excitement become severe.

   4.7. Syndrome of simultaneous manic and depressive responses
   5.2. Phobic and obsessive-compulsive syndromes
   6.5. Affective type of organic brain syndrome

6.6.3.1. Acute schizophrenia-like paranoid-hallucinatory
  syndrome
6.6.3.2. Chronic paranoid syndrome (epileptic)
  6.7. Post-traumatic cerebral syndromes
  6.8. Degenerative brain disorder syndromes
  7.1. Drug abuse syndrome
  7.3. Alcohol induced delirium syndrome
  8.1. Hyperkinetic syndrome (MBD, minimal brain
  dysfunction)
  8.4. Syndrome of periodic episodes of disturbed behavior
  8.5. Autistic child syndrome
  8.6. Infantile juvenile schizophrenic syndromes

Dosage. Outpatient: 50–300 mg; inpatient: 200–900 mg. A double-
blind trial showed that dosages of 100 mg are more effective than 50
mg daily (238).

LEVOMEPROMAZINE/METHOTRIMEPRAZINE (69)

Action. Strongly sedative and anxiolytic, mild antipsychotic, analgesic.

Indications. Anxiety, tension, sleeplessness, psychotic agitation,
pain (carcinoma, herpes zoster, trigeminal neuralgia). The drug is
widely used in Europe but in the U.S. is not yet on the market. The
rather weak antipsychotic effect frequently requires combination
with a piperazine-phenothiazine. Some believe the substance also to
be a mild antidepressant, indicated in the agitated depressive syndrome (39, 61).

Syndromes for which indicated

Primary
  4.2. Agitated depressive syndrome
  4.5. Depressive syndrome with delusions and hallucinations
  4.6. Manic-hypomanic syndrome

5.1. Anxiety state or syndrome
5.2.2. Anoretic syndrome
5.5. Hysterical syndrome
5.5.1. Ganser's syndrome
7.5. Withdrawal syndromes

Also of use in syndromes when marked sedative-anxiolytic and analgesic action is indicated.

Secondary
Useful for sedation in combination with more potent
    antipsychotic drugs
Particularly helpful in intermittent agitated episodes when
    patient is on long term nonsedative antipsychotic treatment
Excellent supplement or replacement for traditional hypnotics

Tolerance. It is a strong sedative, a well-tolerated compound. The main side effect is hypotension.

Special caution. Patients with cardiovascular disorders.

Dosage. Outpatient: 2–50 mg; inpatient: 25–500 mg.

12.2.2. Piperazinylalcyl-phenothiazines

PERPHENAZINE (86)

Action. Strong antipsychotic action without much sedation. The first piperazinylalcyl-phenothiazine on the market. Widely used.

Indications. Hallucinations, delusions, primary thought disorders, mild anxiety, and possibly mild depression. Some authors think that perphenazine also has some antidepressant activity. The preparation is said to be stimulant, activating (125,138,184), or disinhibiting (184,221,223). As a consequence there are combinations of perphenazine with amitriptyline on the market: Triptafon (U.K.), Triavil and Etrafon (U.S.). There are combinations of 25 mg amitriptyline + 2 mg perphenazine and 10 mg amitriptyline + 2 mg perphenazine

(Triptafon–minor). This drug is given in depressive and anxiety syndromes, psychosomatic disorders, and anergic schizophrenic syndromes. Extrapyramidal side effects are milder with a combination of the two drugs.

Syndromes for which indicated

Primary
- **2.1.** Passive paranoid schizophrenic syndrome
- **2.2.** Florid paranoid agitated syndrome
- **2.3.** Systematic paranoid syndrome
- **2.4.** Catatonic schizophrenic syndrome
- **2.5.** Simple schizophrenic syndrome
- **2.6.** Hebephrenic schizophrenic syndrome
- **2.7.** Schizophrenic withdrawal syndrome
- **3.1.** Manic-schizophrenic syndrome
- **3.2.** Depressive-schizophrenic syndrome
- **4.5.** Depressive syndrome with delusions and hallucinations
- **4.6.** Manic-hypomanic syndrome
- **4.7.** Syndrome of simultaneous manic and depressive responses
- **6.6.3.1.** Acute schizophrenia-like paranoid-hallucinatory syndrome
- **6.6.3.2.** Chronic paranoid syndrome (epileptic)
- **6.8.** Degenerative and demyelinating brain disorder syndrome
- **7.4.** Paranoid and hallucinatory syndromes secondary to toxicomania
- **8.5.** Autistic child syndrome
- **8.6.** Infantile juvenile schizophrenic syndromes

Secondary
- **4.2.** Agitated depressive syndrome
- **7.5.** Withdrawal syndromes

Also of use as replacement if tolerance develops or there is danger of dependence on minor tranquilizers.

Contraindications.   Leukopenia, congestive heart failure, coronary artery disease.

Tolerance.   The piperazinylalcyl-phenothiazine derivatives in general have more extrapyramidal activity than drugs with an aliphatic side chain.

Dosage.   Outpatient: 4–48 mg; inpatient: 12–96 mg.

PERPHENAZINE–ENANTHATE

The depot preparation perphenazine-enanthate is not yet on the market.

Indications.   Maintenance treatment of various schizophrenic syndromes.

Syndromes for which indicated

Primary
   2.1. Passive paranoid schizophrenic syndrome
   2.2. Florid paranoid schizophrenic syndrome
   2.3. Systematic paranoid syndrome
   2.4. Catatonic schizophrenic syndrome
   2.5. Simple schizophrenic syndrome
   2.6. Hebephrenic schizophrenic syndrome
   2.7. Schizophrenic withdrawal syndrome
   3.1. Manic-schizophrenic syndrome
   3.2. Depressive schizophrenic syndrome

Secondary
      None

      Of particular use in patients who may not adhere to the recommended regimen.

Dosage.   100 mg i.m. at intervals of two weeks; the effect is the same as with the oral daily application (8a).

FLUPHENAZINE DIHYDROCHLORIDE (47)

Action. Nonsedative, strong major tranquilizer.

Indications. Acute and chronic schizophrenic syndromes, long-term medication. One of the most widely used antipsychotics, at least twelve million patients had been treated with it as of 1968 (19). Acute psychotic syndromes respond better than chronic ones (163).

Syndromes for which indicated

Primary

2.1. Pasive paranoid schizophrenic syndrome
2.2. Florid paranoid agitated syndrome
2.3. Systematic paranoid syndrome
2.4. Catatonic schizophrenic syndrome
2.5. Simple schizophrenic syndrome
2.6. Hebephrenic withdrawal syndrome
2.7. Schizophrenic withdrawal syndrome
3.1. Manic-schizophrenic syndrome
3.2. Depressive schizophrenic syndrome
4.5. Depressive syndrome with delusions and hallucinations
4.6. Manic-hypomanic syndrome
4.7. Syndrome of simultaneous manic and depressive responses
6.6.3.1. Acute schizophrenia-like paranoid-hallucinatory syndrome
6.6.3.2. Chronic parandoid syndrome (epileptic)
6.8. Degenerative and demyelinating brain disorder syndrome
7.4. Paranoid and hallucinatory syndromes secondary to toxicomania
8.5. Autistic child syndrome
8.6. Infantile juvenile schizophrenic syndromes

Secondary

4.2. Agitated depressive syndrome
7.5. Withdrawal syndromes

Also of use as replacement if tolerance develops or there is danger of dependence on minor tranquilizers.

Contraindications. Pheochromocytoma, renal or liver failure, marked cerebral atherosclerosis or severe cardiac insufficiency.

Oral dosage. Outpatient: 1–25 mg or more; inpatient: 2–60 mg or more; children: 0.25–0.5 mg.

Parenteral dosage. 12.5–25 mg or more. The dosage has to be adapted very individually. According to the literature the dosage is very variable and shows a wide range (up to 1500 mg). In therapy-resistant cases 150–300 mg i.m. has been useful (52). A double-blind study showed that daily dosages of 30–60 mg are more effective than low dosages of 7 mg (109). The same has been shown for 800 mg daily compared to 30 mg. Some authors also recommend infusion and believe it leads to better tolerance (54).

Fluphenazine has been combined with tricyclic antidepressants for the treatment of depressive or depressive-schizophrenic syndrome. In Great Britain there is a combination of fluphenazine hydrochloride 0.5 mg with nortriptyline 10 mg on the market (Motival). The dosage is 1–4 tablets daily. It is not recommended for children. This drug is contraindicated in grandmal epilepsy, in subcortical brain damage, and during administration of MAOIs. Special caution is necessary in glaucoma, pregnancy, and urinary retention.

FLUPHENAZINE DECANOATE (46)

Action. Long-term preparation with an action of two to four weeks.

Indications. Maintenance treatment of various schizophrenic syndromes.

Syndromes for which indicated

Primary
    2.1. Passive paranoid schizophrenic syndrome

2.2. Florid paranoid agitated syndrome
2.3. Systematic paranoid syndrome
2.4. Catatonic schizophrenic syndrome
2.5. Simple schizophrenic syndrome
2.6. Hebephrenic withdrawal syndrome
2.7. Schizophrenic withdrawal syndrome
3.1. Manic-schizophrenic syndrome
3.2. Depressive-schizophrenic syndrome

Secondary
None

Of particular use in patients who may not adhere to the recommended regimen. Possibly fewer extrapyramidal side effects and longer action than fluphenazine enanthate.

Contraindication. See fluphenazine dihydrochloride.

Special caution. Persistent extrapyramidal reactions. Antiparkinsonian drugs may be indicated simultaneously. It is recommended to give elderly females only half the normal dose. It is one of the most widely used depot preparations for the outpatient treatment of chronic schizophrenic syndrome (for prevention of relapse and readmission to hospital). The tolerance is better than that of fluphenazine-enanthate and the action is longer.

Dosage. 25–75 mg deep i.m. It is recommended to start the treatment with oral medication or with a dose of 12.5 mg i.m. to test likelihood of extrapyramidal reactions.

FLUPHENAZINE-ENANTHATE (48)

Action. Long-term preparation with an action lasting two to three weeks.

Indications. Maintenance treatment of various schizophrenic syndromes.

Syndromes for which indicated

Primary

    2.1. Passive paranoid schizophrenic syndrome
    2.2. Florid paranoid agitated syndrome
    2.3. Systematic paranoid syndrome
    2.4. Catatonic schizophrenic syndrome
    2.5. Simple schizophrenic syndrome
    2.6. Hebephrenic schizophrenic syndrome
    2.7. Schizophrenic withdrawal syndrome
    3.1. Manic-schizophrenic syndrome
    3.2. Depressive-schizophrenic syndrome

Secondary
    None

Contraindication and special caution.   Pheochromocytoma, renal or liver failure, marked cerebral arteriosclerosis or severe cardiac insufficiency.

Tolerance.   Extrapyramidal side effects seem to be more frequent than during treatment with fluphenazine decanoate.

Dosage.   25 mg i.m. or more at intervals of two weeks.

BUTAPERAZINE (7)

Action.   Very strong major tranquilizer with strong extrapyramidal activity.

Indications.   Acute and chronic florid paranoid agitated schizophrenic syndromes, hallucinations, delusions, motor agitation, and aggression.

Syndromes for which indicated

Primary

    2.1. Passive paranoid schizophrenic syndrome
    2.2. Florid paranoid agitated syndrome
    2.3. Systematic paranoid syndrome
    2.4. Catatonic schizophrenic syndrome

2.5. Simple schizophrenic syndrome

2.6. Hebephrenic schizophrenic syndrome

2.7. Schizophrenic withdrawal syndrome

3.1. Manic-schizophrenic syndrome

3.2. Depressive-schizophrenic syndrome

4.5. Depressive syndrome with delusions and hallucinations

4.6. Manic-hypomanic syndrome

4.7. Syndrome of simultaneous manic and depressive responses

6.6.3.1. Acute schizophrenia-like paranoid-hallucinatory syndrome

6.6.3.2. Chronic paranoid syndrome (epileptic)

6.8. Degenerative and demyelinating brain disorder syndromes

7.4. Paranoid and hallucinatory syndromes secondary to toxicomania

8.5. Autistic child syndrome

8.6. Infantile juvenile schizophrenic syndromes

Secondary

4.2. Agitated depressive syndrome

7.5. Withdrawal syndromes

Also of use as replacement if tolerance develops or there is danger of dependence on minor tranquilizers.

Tolerance. Strong extrapyramidal activity.

Dosage. Outpatient: 10–30 mg; inpatient: 10–100 mg. A very well controlled study by Simpson and coworkers (214) compared four grades of dosages (5–40, 40–80, 80–120, 120–160 mg per day). It seems that in some patients lower dosages are a bit more effective, and the conclusion is that the dosage has to be adapted individually. There are no general rules.

THIOPROPAZATE (123)

Action. Nonsedative, strong major tranquilizer.

Indications. Schizophrenic syndromes. The drug has been especially recommended for the treatment of catatonic syndromes, for catatonic stupor, and anergia. This is especially true for a combination of thiopropazate with a central stimulant and antiparkinson drug. It is recommended for daily long-term treatment.

Syndromes for which indicated

Primary
2.1. Passive paranoid schizophrenic syndrome
2.2. Florid paranoid agitated syndrome
2.3. Systematic paranoid syndrome
2.4. Catatonic schizophrenic syndrome
2.5. Simple schizophrenic syndrome
2.6. Hebephrenic schizophrenic syndrome
2.7. Schizophrenic withdrawal syndrome
3.1. Manic-schizophrenic syndrome
3.2. Depressive-schizophrenic syndrome
4.5. Depressive syndrome with delusions and hallucinations
4.6. Manic-hypomanic syndrome
4.7. Syndrome of simultaneous manic and depressive responses
6.6.3.1. Acute schizophrenia-like paranoid-hallucinatory syndrome
6.6.3.2. Chronic paranoid syndrome (epileptic)
6.8. Degenerative and demyelinating brain disorder syndromes
7.4. Paranoid and hallucinatory syndromes secondary to toxicomania
8.5. Autistic child syndrome
8.6. Infantile juvenile schizophrenic syndromes

Secondary
4.2. Agitated depressive syndrome
7.5. Withdrawal syndromes

Also of use as replacement if tolerance develops or there is danger of dependence on minor tranquilizers.

Dosage.   Outpatient: 10–30 mg; inpatient: 30–60 mg.

TRIFLUOPERAZINE (130)

Action. Nonsedative, strong major tranquilizer. Many authors thought that the drug should be more activating or more antiautistic than others, but double-blind trials did not show significant differences. It is one of the most widely used drugs for the treatment of schizophrenic syndromes in Western and Eastern countries.

Indications. Acute and chronic schizophrenic syndromes, hallucinations, autism, anergia, delusions. The drug has also been applied in the treatment of children. It has been especially recommended for the treatment of chronic schizophrenic syndromes and shown to be very useful even after treatment for more than 9 years (95). A combination with chlorpromazine has been recommended for florid paranoid agitated schizophrenic syndromes (14, 152, 155, 224).

Syndromes for which indicated

Primary
  2.1. Passive paranoid schizophrenic syndrome
  2.2. Florid paranoid agitated syndrome
  2.3. Systematic paranoid syndrome
  2.4. Catatonic schizophrenic syndrome
  2.5. Simple schizophrenic syndrome
  2.6. Hebephrenic schizophrenic syndrome
  2.7. Schizophrenic withdrawal syndrome
  3.1. Manic-schizophrenic syndrome
  3.2. Depressive-schizophrenic syndrome
  4.5. Depressive syndrome with delusions and hallucinations
  4.6. Manic-hypomanic syndrome
  4.7. Syndrome of simultaneous manic and depressive responses
6.6.3.1. Acute schizophrenia-like paranoid-hallucinatory syndrome
6.6.3.2. Chronic paranoid syndrome (epileptic)
  6.8. Degenerative and demyelinating brain disorder syndromes
  7.4. Paranoid and hallucinatory syndromes secondary to toxicomania

8.5. Austitic child syndrome
8.6. Infantile juvenile schizophrenic syndromes

Secondary
4.2. Agitated depressive syndrome
7.5. Withdrawal syndromes

Also of use as a replacement if tolerance develops or there is a danger of dependence on minor tranquilizers.

Contraindications. Blood dyscrasias, bone marrow depression and preexisting liver damage.

Tolerance. In a double-blind trial autonomic withdrawal symptoms (rebound) have been observed manifested by nausea and vomiting (76).

Dosage. Outpatient: 4–20 mg; inpatient: 6–40 mg. The drug can be given once a day (181). The question whether high doses are more effective than lower dosages is controversial. (38, 44, 175).

PROCHLORPERAZINE (95)

Action: Nonsedative major tranquilizer. The action is similar to other good major tranquilizers.

Indications. Acute and chronic schizophrenic syndromes.

Syndromes for which indicated

Primary
2.1. Passive paranoid schizophrenic syndrome
2.2. Florid paranoid agitated syndrome
2.3. Systematic paranoid syndrome
2.4. Catatonic schizophrenic syndrome
2.5. Simple schizophrenic syndrome
2.6. Hebephrenic schizophrenic syndrome
2.7. Schizophrenic withdrawal syndrome
3.1. Manic-schizophrenic syndrome
3.2. Depressive-schizophrenic syndrome
4.5. Depressive syndrome with delusions and hallucinations

4.6. Manic-hypomanic syndrome

4.7. Syndrome of simultaneous manic and depressive responses

6.6.3.1. Acute schizophrenia-like paranoid-hallucinatory syndrome

6.6.3.2. Chronic paranoid syndrome (epileptic)

6.8. Degenerative and demyelinating brain disorder syndrome

7.4. Paranoid and hallucinatory syndromes secondary to toxicomania

8.5. Autistic child syndrome

8.6. Infantile juvenile schizophrenic syndromes

Secondary

4.2. Agitated depressive syndrome

7.5. Withdrawal syndromes

Also of use as replacement if tolerance develops or there is danger of dependence on minor tranquilizers.

Contraindication. Undiagnosed and prolonged vomiting.

Dosage. Outpatient: 15–120 mg; inpatient: 30–150 mg; long-term: 15 mg daily.

ACETOPHENAZINE (4)

Action. Nonsedative major tranquilizer.

Indications. Acute and chronic schizophrenic syndromes, adults and children (see 104, 159, 190).

Syndromes for which indicated

Primary

2.1. Passive paranoid schizophrenic syndrome

2.2. Florid paranoid agitated syndrome

2.3. Systematic paranoid syndrome

2.4. Catatonic schizophrenic syndrome

2.5. Simple schizophrenic syndrome

2.6. Hebephrenic schizophrenic syndrome
2.7. Schizophrenic withdrawal syndrome
3.1. Manic-schizophrenic syndrome
3.2. Depressive-schizophrenic syndrome
4.5. Depressive syndrome with delusions and hallucinations
4.6. Manic-hypomanic syndrome
4.7. Syndrome of simultaneous manic and depressive responses
6.6.3.1. Acute schizophrenia-like paranoid-hallucinatory syndrome
6.6.3.2. Chronic paranoid syndrome (epileptic)
7.4. Paranoid and hallucinatory syndromes secondary to toxicomania
8.5. Autistic child syndrome
8.6. Infantile juvenile schizophrenic syndromes

Secondary
4.2. Agitated depressive syndrome
7.5. Withdrawal syndromes

Also of use as replacement if tolerance develops or there is danger of dependence on minor tranquilizers.

Dosage. Outpatient: 40–60 mg; inpatient: 60–80 mg.

CARPHENAZINE (9)

Action. Nonsedative major tranquilizer.

Indications. Some authors recommend carphenazine especially for chronic therapy-resistant schizophrenic syndromes and for outpatients in need of long-term treatment (48, 88). The action is very similar to chlorpromazine and trifluoperazine (165, 219). It has also been recommended for anergic apathetic states (31, 188, 189).

Syndromes for which indicated

Primary
2.1. Passive paranoid schizophrenic syndrome
2.2. Florid paranoid agitated syndrome

2.3. Systematic paranoid syndrome
2.4. Catatonic schizophrenic syndrome
2.5. Simple schizophrenic syndrome
2.6. Hebephrenic schizophrenic syndrome
2.7. Schizophrenic withdrawal syndrome
3.1. Manic-schizophrenic syndrome
3.2. Depressive-schizophrenic syndrome
4.5. Depressive syndrome with delusions and hallucinations
4.6. Manic-hypomanic syndrome
4.7. Syndrome of simultaneous manic and depressive responses
6.6.3.1. Acute schizophrenia-like paranoid-hallucinatory syndrome
6.6.3.2. Chronic paranoid syndrome (epileptic)
7.4. Paranoid and hallucinatory syndromes secondary to toxicomania
8.5. Autistic child syndrome
8.6. Infantile juvenile schizophrenic syndromes

Secondary
4.2. Agitated depressive syndrome
7.5. Withdrawal syndromes

Also of use as replacement if tolerance develops or there is danger of dependence on minor tranquilizers.

Tolerance. The same as other piperazine-phenothiazines.

Dosage. Outpatient: 25–200 mg; inpatient: 50–400 mg.

12.2.3. Piperidylalcyl-phenothiazines

THIORIDAZINE (125)

Action. Mild sedative, moderate antipsychotic action, anxiolytic, perhaps slight antidepressive.

Indications. Chronic and mild acute schizophrenic syndromes, anxiety, tension, agitated depression, senile agitation, behavior disorders in children. Thioridazine is one of the most widely used major tranquilizers in the world. It has been particularly recommended for outpatient and long-term treatment.

Syndromes for which indicated

Primary
- **2.1.** Passive paranoid schizophrenic syndrome
- **2.3.** Systematic paranoid syndrome
- **2.4.** Catatonic schizophrenic syndrome
- **2.5.** Simple schizophrenic syndrome
- **2.6.** Hebephrenic schizophrenic syndrome
- **2.7.** Schizophrenic withdrawal syndrome
- **3.2.** Depressive-schizophrenic syndrome
- **4.1.** Retarded depressive syndrome
- **4.2.** Agitated depressive syndrome
- **4.3.** Affective hypochondriacal syndrome
- **4.4.** Depressed obsessive-compulsive syndrome
- **4.5.** Depressive syndrome with delusions and hallucinations
- **6.6.3.1.** Acute schizophrenia-like paranoid-hallucinatory syndrome
- **6.6.3.2.** Chronic paranoid syndrome (epileptic)
- **7.4.** Paranoid and hallucinatory syndromes secondary to toxicomania

Secondary
- **5.1.** Anxiety state or syndrome
- **5.2.** Phobic and obsessive-compulsive syndromes
- **5.3.** Depressive neurotic syndrome
- **5.4.** Neurotic hypochondriacal syndrome
- **6.5.** Affective type of organic brain syndrome
- **6.7.** Post-traumatic cerebral syndromes
- **6.8.** Degenerative and demyelinating brain disorder syndromes
- **8.5.** Autistic child syndrome
- **8.6.** Infantile juvenile schizophrenic syndromes
- **9.** Oligophrenic syndrome

Tolerance. Thioridazine is generally very well tolerated.

Dosage. Outpatient: 75–400 mg; inpatient: 200–800 mg. Keep the long-term dosage as low as possible because of side effects (EKG, pigmentation).

PIPERACETAZINE (93)

Action. Nonsedative major tranquilizer.

Indications. The drug is more effective in acute than in chronic schizophrenic syndromes (13). It can be used as other major tranquilizers. Some authors stress a quick onset of action (22).

Syndromes for which indicated

Primary

2.1. Passive paranoid schizophrenic syndrome
2.2. Florid paranoid agitated syndrome
2.3. Systematic paranoid syndrome
2.4. Catatonic schizophrenic syndrome
2.5. Simple schizophrenic syndrome
2.6. Hebephrenic schizophrenic syndrome
2.7. Schizophrenic withdrawal syndrome
3.1. Manic-schizophrenic syndrome
3.2. Depressive-schizophrenic syndrome
4.5. Depressive syndrome with delusions and hallucinations
4.6. Manic-hypomanic syndrome
4.7. Syndrome of simultaneous manic and depressive responses
6.6.3.1. Acute schizophrenia-like paranoid-hallucinatory syndrome
6.6.3.2. Chronic paranoid syndrome (epileptic)
7.4. Paranoid and hallucinatory syndromes secondary to toxicomania
8.5. Autistic child syndrome
8.6. Infantile juvenile schizophrenic syndromes

Secondary

4.2. Agitated depressive syndrome
7.5. Withdrawal syndromes

Also of use as replacement if tolerance develops or there is a danger of dependence on minor tranquilizers.

Tolerance. Good.

Dosage. Outpatient; 10–40 mg; inpatient: 20–160 mg. Daily dosages of 400 mg are more effective than 150 mg (75).

MESORIDAZINE (65)

Action. Strong sedative and good antipsychotic, perhaps also slightly antidepressant. The drug gives rapid sedation and subsequent antipsychotic effect.

Indications. Florid paranoid schizophrenic syndrome (hallucinations, paranoid delusions), tension, agitation, anxiety, agitated depression. The drug can be used with children.

Syndromes for which indicated

Primary
- **2.1.** Passive paranoid schizophrenic syndrome
- **2.3.** Systematic paranoid syndrome
- **2.4.** Catatonic schizophrenic syndrome
- **2.5.** Simple schizophrenic syndrome
- **2.6.** Hebephrenic schizophrenic syndrome
- **2.7.** Schizophrenic withdrawal syndrome
- **3.2.** Depressive-schizophrenic syndrome
- **4.1.** Retarded depressive syndrome
- **4.2.** Agitated depressive syndrome
- **4.3.** Affective hypochondriacal syndrome
- **4.4.** Depressed obsessive-compulsive syndrome
- **4.5.** Depressive syndrome with delusions and hallucinations
- **6.6.3.1.** Acute schizophrenia-like paranoid-hallucinatory syndrome
- **6.6.3.2.** Chronic paranoid syndrome (epileptic)
- **7.4.** Paranoid and hallucinatory syndromes secondary to toxicomania

Secondary
- **5.1.** Anxiety state or syndrome
- **5.2.** Phobic and obsessive-compulsive syndromes
- **5.3.** Depressive neurotic syndrome
- **5.4.** Neurotic hypochondriacal syndrome
- **6.5.** Affective type of organic brain syndrome
- **6.7.** Post-traumatic cerebral syndromes
- **6.8.** Degenerative and demyelinating brain disorder syndromes
- **8.5.** Autistic child syndrome
- **8.6.** Infantile juvenile schizophrenic syndromes
- **9.** Oligophrenic syndrome

Tolerance. Good.

Dosage. Outpatient; 75–400 mg; inpatient: 150–600 mg.

PROPERICIAZINE (100)

Action. Mild sedative, moderate major tranquilizer.

Indications. Acute and chronic schizophrenic cases, behavioral and character disorders, anxiety and tension, agitation, aggression.

Syndromes for which indicated

Primary
- **2.1.** Passive paranoid schizophrenic syndrome
- **2.3.** Systematic paranoid syndrome
- **2.4.** Catatonic schizophrenic syndrome
- **2.5.** Simple schizophrenic syndrome
- **2.6.** Hebephrenic schizophrenic syndrome
- **2.7.** Schizophrenic withdrawal syndrome
- **3.2.** Depressive-schizophrenic syndrome
- **5.5.** Hysterical syndrome
- **5.5.1.** Ganser's syndrome
- **5.6.** Neurasthenic syndrome
- **5.7.** Sexual neurotic syndrome

6.6.3.1. Acute schizophrenia-like paranoid-hallucinatory syndrome

6.6.3.2. Chronic paranoid syndrome (epileptic)

7.4. Paranoid and hallucinatory syndromes secondary to toxicomania

8.5. Autistic child syndrome

8.6. Infantile juvenile schizophrenic syndromes

9. Oligophrenic syndrome

Secondary

4.1. Retarded depressive syndrome

4.2. Agitated depressive syndrome

4.3. Affective hypochondriacal syndrome

4.4. Depressed obsessive-compulsive syndrome

5.1. Anxiety state or syndrome

Tolerance. Good, side effects are strongly dose related.

Dosage. Outpatient: 10–60 mg; inpatient: 50–500 mg. In low dosages the sedative effect is rather mild, in high dosages strong. Also for use with children (78).

12.2.4. Azaphenothiazine derivatives

PROTHIPENDYL (938)

Action. Sedative, perhaps antipsychotic (215).

Indications. Anxiety, agitation, insomnia, nausea, vomiting.

Syndromes for which indicated

Primary

4.2. Agitated depressive syndrome

5.1. Anxiety state or syndrome

5.2. Phobic and obsessive-compulsive syndromes

5.3. Depressive neurotic syndrome

Secondary

None

Special caution.   Susceptibility to orthostatic hypotension.

Dosage.   Outpatient: 40–120 mg; inpatient: 40–300 mg.

12.3. Thioxanthene derivatives

CHLORPROTHIXENE (168)

Action.   Sedative, sleep inducing, moderate antipsychotic, perhaps antidepressant.

Indications.   Agitated depression, anxiety states, sleeplessness in psychoses and neuroses, aggression.

Syndromes for which indicated

Primary
- **2.2.** Florid paranoid agitated syndrome
- **2.6.** Hebephrenic schizophrenic syndrome
- **2.7.** Schizophrenic withdrawal syndrome
- **3.2.** Depressive-schizophrenic syndrome
- **4.1.** Retarded depressive syndrome
- **4.2.** Agitated depressive syndrome
- **4.3.** Affective hypochondriacal syndrome
- **4.5.** Depressive syndrome with delusions and hallucinations
- **4.6.** Manic-hypomanic syndrome
- **4.7.** Syndrome of simultaneous manic and depressive responses
- **5.1.** Anxiety state or syndrome
- **5.4.** Neurotic hypochondriacal syndrome
- **5.5.** Hysterical syndrome
- **5.5.1.** Ganser's syndrome
- **9.** Oligophrenic syndrome

Secondary
- **2.1.** Passive paranoid schizophrenic syndrome
- **2.3.** Systematic paranoid syndrome
- **2.4.** Catatonic schizophrenic syndrome
- **2.5.** Simple schizophrenic syndrome
- **6.5.** Affective type of organic brain syndrome

6.7. Post-traumatic cerebral syndromes
6.8. Degenerative and demyelinating brain disorder syndromes
8.5. Autistic child syndrome
8.6. Infantile juvenile schizophrenic syndromes

Tolerance. Only very mild extrapyramidal activity, more frequent autonomic side effects.

Dosage. Outpatient: 30–300 mg; inpatient 75–600 mg.

CLOPENTHIXOL (173)

Action. Strong sedative and antipsychotic, anxiolytic.

Indications. Florid paranoid agitated schizophrenic syndrome, manic syndrome, aggression and anxiety of various etiology.

Syndromes for which indicated

Primary
2.2. Florid paranoid agitated syndrome
2.3. Systematic paranoid syndrome
2.4. Catatonic schizophrenic syndrome
2.6. Hebephrenic schizophrenic syndrome
3.1. Manic-schizophrenic syndrome
4.6. Manic-hypomanic syndrome
4.7. Syndrome of simultaneous manic and depressive responses
6.6.3.1. Acute schizophrenia-like paranoid-hallucinatory syndrome
6.6.3.2. Chronic paranoid syndrome (epileptic)
7.4. Paranoid and hallucinatory syndromes secondary to toxicomania
8.6. Infantile juvenile schizophrenic syndromes

Secondary
4.2. Agitated depressive syndrome
5.1. Anxiety state or syndrome

Tolerance. In high doses oversedation, autonomic side effects.

Dosage. Outpatient: 15–150 mg; inpatient: 75–500 mg.

FLUPENTHIXOL (191)

Action. Nonsedative antipsychotic.

Indications. Anergia, autism, retardation, apathy, depression, anxiety states, obsessive-compulsive neurotic syndromes.

Syndromes for which indicated

Primary
- **2.1.** Passive paranoid schizophrenic syndrome
- **2.3.** Systematic paranoid syndrome
- **2.4.** Catatonic schizophrenic syndrome
- **2.5.** Simple schizophrenic syndrome
- **2.6.** Hebephrenic schizophrenic syndrome
- **2.7.** Schizophrenic withdrawal syndrome
- **3.2.** Depressive-schizophrenic syndrome
- **4.4.** Depressed obsessive-compulsive syndrome
- **4.5.** Depressive syndrome with delusions and hallucinations
- **6.6.3.1.** Acute schizophrenia-like paranoid-hallucinatory syndrome
- **6.6.3.2.** Chronic paranoid syndrome (epileptic)
- **7.4.** Paranoid and hallucinatory syndromes secondary to toxicomania
- **7.5.** Autistic child syndrome
- **7.6.** Infantile juvenile schizophrenic syndromes

Secondary
- **4.1.** Retarded depressive syndrome
- **5.1.** Anxiety state or syndrome
- **5.2.** Phobic and obsessive-compulsive syndromes
- **5.3.** Depressive neurotic syndrome
- **6.5.** Affective type of organic brain syndrome
- **6.7.** Post-traumatic cerebral syndromes
- **6.8.** Degenerative and demyelinating brain disorder syndromes

Tolerance. Relatively good.

Dosage. Outpatient: 1.5–4.5. mg; inpatient: 1.5–30 mg.

FLUPENTHIXOL DECANOATE

Action. As flupenthixol, long-term preparation.

Indications. In anergic schizophrenic conditions.

Syndromes for which indicated

Primary
> **2.1.** Passive paranoid schizophrenic syndrome
> **2.3.** Systematic paranoid syndrome
> **2.4.** Catatonic schizophrenic syndrome
> **2.5.** Simple schizophrenic syndrome
> **2.6.** Hebephrenic schizophrenic syndrome
> **2.7.** Schizophrenic withdrawal syndrome

Secondary
> None

Tolerance. Relatively good.

Dosage. 20–40mg i.m. at intervals of two to four weeks.

THIOTHIXENE (243)

Action. Nonsedative major tranquilizer, activating.

Indications Chronic schizophrenic states, withdrawal, apathy, inhibition, anergia, loss of contact, long-term medication for rehabilitation, anxiety and depressive states, particularly schizoaffective syndromes.

Syndromes for which indicated

Primary
> **2.1.** Passive paranoid schizophrenic syndrome
> **2.3.** Systematic paranoid syndrome

2.4. Catatonic schizophrenic syndrome

2.5. Simple schizophrenic syndrome

2.6. Hebephrenic schizophrenic syndrome

2.7. Schizophrenic withdrawal syndrome

3.2. Depressive-schizophrenic syndrome

4.1. Retarded depressive syndrome

4.4. Depressed obsessive-compulsive syndrome

4.5. Depressive syndrome with delusions and hallucinations

4.7. Syndrome of simultaneous manic and depressive responses

5.1. Anxiety state or syndrome

5.3. Depressive neurotic syndrome

5.6. Neurasthenic syndrome

6.6.3.1. Acute schizophrenia-like paranoid-hallucinatory syndrome

6.6.3.2. Chronic paranoid syndrome (epileptic)

8.3. Unmotivated retarded child syndrome

8.5. Autistic child syndrome

Secondary
> None

Side effects. More extrapyramidal than autonomic.

Dosage. Outpatient: 6–50 mg; inpatient: 10–100 mg; children: 1–10 mg.

12.4. Butyrophenones

The butyrophenones in general have actions very similar to the phenothiazines, as has been shown by many double-blind studies. They have strong extrapyramidal activity.

HALOPERIDOL (621)

Action. Sedative, antipsychotic.

Indications Acute and chronic schizophrenic syndromes, manic syndromes, agitation of different etiologies.

Syndromes for which indicated

Primary
2.1. Passive paranoid schizophrenic syndrome
2.2. Florid paranoid agitated syndrome
2.3. Systematic paranoid syndrome
2.4. Catatonic schizophrenic syndrome
2.5. Simple schizophrenic syndrome
2.6. Hebephrenic schizophrenic syndrome
2.7. Schizophrenic withdrawal syndrome
3.1. Manic-schizophrenic syndrome
3.2. Depressive-schizophrenic syndrome
4.6. Manic-hypomanic syndrome
4.7. Syndrome of simultaneous manic and depressive responses
5.2.1. Gilles de la Tourette syndrome
6.6.3.1. Acute schizophrenia-like paranoid-hallucinatory syndrome
6.6.3.2. Chronic paranoid syndrome (epileptic)
6.8. Degenerative and demyelinating brain disorder syndromes
7.4. Paranoid and hallucinatory syndromes secondary to toxicomania
8.5. Autistic child syndrome
8.6. Infantile juvenile schizophrenic syndrome
9. Oligophrenic syndrome

Secondary
4.2. Agitated depressive syndrome
4.5. Depressive syndrome with delusions and hallucinations
5.1. Anxiety state or syndrome

Special caution.   May accentuate parkinsonism and other extrapyramidal symptoms.

Dosage.   Outpatient: 2–60 mg; inpatient: 4–80 mg.

TRIFLUPERIDOL (633)

Action.   At low doses not sedative, at high doses sedative and antipsychotic.

Indications. Anergic schizophrenic syndromes, autism, stupor, residual states with withdrawal.

Syndromes for which indicated

Primary
2.1. Passive paranoid schizophrenic syndrome
2.3. Systematic paranoid syndrome
2.4. Catatonic schizophrenic syndrome
2.5. Simple schizophrenic syndrome
2.7. Schizophrenic withdrawal syndrome
3.2. Depressive-schizophrenic syndrome
6.8. Degenerative and demyelinating brain disorder syndromes
8.3. Unmotivated retarded child syndrome
8.5. Autistic child syndrome

Secondary
None

Contraindications. Pregnancy, neurological disorders with extrapyramidal symptoms.

Tolerance. Side effects are dose related (212), marked extrapyramidal effect in higher dosages.

Dosage. 1–10 mg; children: 0.5–3 mg.

BENPERIDOL (608)

Action. Sedative, antipsychotic. One of the stronger butyrophenones (dosage is related to clinical effect).

Indications. Deviant and antisocial sexual behavior; acute schizophrenia, agitation.

Syndromes for which indicated

Primary
2.2. Florid paranoid agitated syndrome
2.4. Catatonic schizophrenic syndrome

5.7. Sexual neurotic syndrome

Secondary
    3.1. Manic-schizophrenic syndrome
    4.6. Manic-hypomanic syndrome

Contraindications.   Pyramidal or extrapyramidal symptoms.

Dosage.   0.25–1.5 mg.

12.5. Diphenylbutylpiperidine

PIMOZIDE (925)

Action.   Nonsedative piperidine derivative with some activating effect.

Indications.   Oral long-term treatment: chronic schizophrenic syndromes, delusions, hallucinations, autism, loss of contact, apathy, inhibition.

Syndromes for which indicated

  Primary
    2.1. Passive paranoid schizophrenic syndrome
    2.3. Systematic paranoid syndrome
    2.4. Catatonic schizophrenic syndrome
    2.5. Simple schizophrenic syndrome
    2.7. Schizophrenic withdrawal syndrome
    3.2. Depressive schizophrenic syndrome
    8.5. Autistic child syndrome
    8.6. Infantile juvenile schizophrenic syndromes

  Secondary
    None

Tolerance.   Relatively good

Dosage.   Outpatient: 3–16 mg; inpatient: 5–20 mg or more. Administration once in twenty-four hours.

FLUSPIRILENE (753)

Action. Injectable long-acting preparation in crystal suspension, antipsychotic.

Indication. Long-term treatment of schizophrenic syndromes.

Syndromes for which indicated.

Primary
   2.2. Florid paranoid agitated syndrome
   2.3. Systematic paranoid syndrome
   2.4. Catatonic schizophrenic syndrome
   2.6. Hebephrenic schizophrenic syndrome
   3.1. Manic-schizophrenic syndrome
   4.6. Manic-hypomanic syndrome

Secondary
   None

Contraindication. Extrapyramidal disorders, endogenous depression, organic brain disorders, epilepsy.

Dosage. Outpatient: 1–3 mg i.m. once a week; inpatient: 2–6 mg i.m. once a week.

PENFLURIDOL (909)

Action. First *oral* long-acting major tranquilizer with about one week action. The development of this drug is a substantial step forward, because the prolonged action does not require intramuscular injections.

Indication. Long-term treatment of schizophrenic syndromes (in- and outpatients). Its possible use in other psychotic syndromes is still under study.

Syndromes for which indicated

Primary
   2.2. Florid paranoid agitated syndrome

2.3. Systematic paranoid syndrome
2.4. Catatonic schizophrenic syndrome
2.6. Hebephrenic schizophrenic syndrome
3.1. Manic-schizophrenic syndrome
4.6. Manic-hypomanic syndrome

Secondary
None

Dosage   20–40 mg once a week.

12.6. Dibenzodiazepine derivatives

CLOZAPINE (199)*

Action.   Initially strong sedative, potent antipsychotic.

Indications.   Acute and chronic schizophrenic syndromes, agitation, aggression, anxiety, hallucinations, manic syndromes, sleep disturbance; sometimes is effective when other antipsychotic agents are unsuccessful. Use when extrapyramidal side effects are not acceptable. May be particularly useful in patients with tardive dyskinesia.

Side Effects.   Leukopenia. Withdrawn from widespread premarket testing because of several deaths. However, appears relatively safe if not reduced WBCs in first 2 months of use. Agranulocytosis develops slowly and seems to be dosage related.

Syndromes for which indicated

Primary
2.1. Passive paranoid schizophrenic syndrome
2.2. Florid paranoid agitated syndrome
2.3. Systematic paranoid agitated syndrome
2.4. Catatonic schizophrenic syndrome
2.5. Simple schizophrenic syndrome
2.6. Hebephrenic schizophrenic syndrome

---

* Because of a possible relationship to agranulocytosis this drug has not been cleared for marketing.

2.7. Schizophrenic withdrawal syndrome
3.1. Manic-schizophrenic syndrome
4.6. Manic-hypomanic syndrome
4.7. Syndrome of simultaneous manic and depressive responses
7.4. Paranoid and hallucinatory syndromes secondary to toxicomania
8.6. Infantile juvenile schizophrenic syndromes
9. Oligophrenic syndrome

Secondary
4.2. Agitated depressive syndrome
5.1. Anxiety state or syndrome
5.4. Neurotic hypochondriacal syndrome
5.5. Hysterical syndrome
5.5.1. Ganser's syndrome

Tolerance. Autonomic side effects, up to now no extrapyramidal side effects observed. Initially may be very sedative (start with low dose). Hypersalivation.

Dosage. Outpatient: 12.5–150 mg; inpatient: 25–600 mg.

12.7. Benzochinolizines (Rauwolfia alkaloids)

RESERPINE (318)

Action. Strongly sedative, potent antipsychotic.

Indications. Acute and chronic schizophrenic syndromes, manic syndromes.

Syndromes for which indicated.

Primary
2.2. Florid paranoid agitated syndrome
2.4. Catatonic schizophrenic syndrome
2.6. Hebephrenic schizophrenic syndrome
3.1. Manic-schizophrenic syndrome
4.6. Manic-hypomanic syndrome

6.8. Degenerative and demyelinating brain disorder syndromes

Secondary
      None

Tolerance.   Initial sedation, marked extrapyramidal side effects; may produce depression, hypotensive action.

Contraindication.   History of gastric or duodenal ulcer. Contraindicated in combination with electroconvulsive treatment (ECT).

Dosage.   Outpatient: 1–3 mg; inpatient: 1–15 mg.

12. Antipsychotic drugs (major tranquilizers)

Generic Name	Trade Name			Usual Dosage
	U.K.	U.S.	Canada	
Phenothiazines				
Aminoalkyl-phenothiazines				
Promazine (98)	Sparine	Sparine	Sparine, Promabec, Promanyl	*o: 25- 600 mg, *i: 150-1000 mg
Chlorpromazine (20)	Chloractil, Largactil	Thorazine	Largactil, Chlorprom, Chlorpromanyl	o: 50-1000 mg, i: 200-2000 mg
Triflupromazine (132) (Flupromazine)		Vesprin	Vesprin	o: 50- 300 mg, i: 200- 900 mg
Levomepromazine/ Methotrimeprazine (69)	Veractil	Levoprome	Nozinan	o: 2- 50 mg, i: 25- 500 mg
Piperazinalcyl-phenothiazines				
Perphenazine (86)	Fentazin	Trilafon	Trilafon, Phenazine	o: 4-48 mg, i: 12-96 mg
Perphenazine-enanthate		not yet on the market		100 mg i.m. at intervals of 2 weeks
Fluphenazine dihydrochloride (47)	Moditen	Permitil, Prolixin	Moditen	o: 1-15 mg, i: 2-20 mg or more children: 0.25-0.5 mg
Fluphenazine decanoate (46)	Modecate	Prolixin decanoate	Modecate	25 (-75) mg deep i.m.
Fluphenazine enanthate (48)	Moditen enanthate	Prolixin enanthate	Moditen enanthate	25 mg i.m. or more at intervals of 2 weeks

*o = outpatient / *i = inpatient

Generic Name	Trade Name			Usual Dosage
	U.K.	U.S.	Canada	
Butaperazine (7)		Repoise		o: 10– 30 mg i: 10–100 mg
Thiopropazate (123)	Dartalan		Dartal	o: 10– 30 mg i: 30– 60 mg
Trifluoperazine (130)	Stelazine	Stelazine	Stelazine Clinazine Novaflurazine Pentazine Solazine Terfluzine Triflurin Tripazine	o: 4– 20 mg i: 6– 40 mg
Prochlorperazine (95)	Stemetil	Compazine	Stemetil	o: 15–120 mg i: 30–150 mg long-term: 15 mg daily
Acetophenazine (4)		Tindal		o: 40– 60 mg i: 60– 80 mg
Carphenazine (9) (Maleate)		Proketazine		o: 25–200 mg i: 50–400 mg
Piperidylalcyl-phenothiazines				
Thioridazine (125)	Melleril	Mellaril	Mellaril Novoridazine Thioril	o: 75–400 mg i: 200–800 mg
Piperacetazine (93)		Quide	Quide	o: 10– 40 mg i: 20–160 mg
Mesoridazine (65)		Serentil	Serentil	o: 75–200 mg i: 150–600 mg
Propericiazine (100) (Pericyazine)	Neulactil		Neuleptil	o: 10– 60 mg i: 50–500 mg

Generic Name	Trade Name			Usual Dosage
	U.K.	U.S.	Canada	
Azaphenothiazine derivatives				
Prothipendyl (938)	Tolnate			o: 40–120 mg i: –300 mg
Thioxanthene derivatives				
Chlorprothixene (168)	Taractan	Taractan	Tarasan	o: 30–300 mg i: 75–600 mg
Clopenthixol (173)	Sordinol: not yet on the market			o: 15–150 mg i: –500 mg
Flupenthixol (191)	Fluanxol			o: 1.5– 4.5 mg i: – 30 mg
Flupenthixol decanoate	Depixol			20–40 mg i.m. at intervals of 2–4 weeks
Thiothixene (243)	Navane	Navane	Navane	o: 6– 60 mg i: 10–100 mg children: 1–10 mg
Butyrophenones				
Haloperidol (621)	Haldol Serenase	Haldol	Haldol	o: 2– 60 mg i: 4– 80 mg
Trifluperidol (633)	Triperidol			1–10 mg children: 0.5–3 mg
Beneperidol (608)	Anquil			0.25–1.5 mg
Diphenylbutylpiperidine				
Pimozide (925)	Orap		Orap	o: 3– 20 mg i: (once within 24 hours)
Fluspirilene (753)	Redeptin		Imap	o: 1– 3 mg i.m. i: 2– 6 mg i.m. (once a week)
Penfluridol (909)	Longoperidol, Semap: not yet on the market			20–40 mg (once a week)

Generic Name	Trade Name			Usual Dosage
	U.K.	U.S.	Canada	
Dibenzodiazepine derivatives				
Clozapine (199)		Leponex: not yet on the market		o: 12.5–150 mg i: 25–600 mg
Benzochinolizines				
Reserpine (318)	Serpasil	Serpasil Demi-Regroton Diupres Diutensen-R Tablets Dralserp Exna-R Tablets Hydromox R Tablets Hydropres Hydrotensin-25 Tablets Hydrotensin-50 Tablets Metatensin Naquival Tablets Rau-Sed Regroton Renese-R Reserpine Tablets Reserpine Tablets, USP SK-Reserpine Tablets Salutensin/Salutensin-Demi Sandril Sandril Tablets Ser-Ap-Es Serpasil Parenteral Solution Serpasil Tablets, Elixir Serpasil-Apresoline Serpasil-Esidrix	Serpasil Neo-serp Reserfia Reserpanca	o: 1–3 mg i: 1– 15 mg

13. ANTIDEPRESSANTS

13.1. Definition

Depression as a syndrome is the consequence of various pathological processes. The syndromes may be characterized by several of the following symptoms: loss of interests, indecision, reduced capacity for enjoyment, reduced productivity. The mood is depressed, sad or indifferent, accompanied by inner restlessness, feelings of anxiety, loss of energy, drive, motor activity. Speech may be slow, retarded, low. The capacity for thinking is burdened with depressive contents, ideas of guilt, hypochondriasis, and delusions of poverty.

13.2. Principles of treatment

Treatment of depression should include clear instructions to the patient and his relatives as to the nature of the disorder, the necessity and prospects of treatment, and the side effects and time-lag for effectiveness of most drugs (usually three weeks). Retarded depressed patients need also to be relieved as far as possible from unnecessary responsibility and stress. The dosage should be increased unless side effects become too serious or until response is observed. Many patients are undertreated with low dosages (e.g., less than 100 mg of a tricyclic/tetracyclic antidepressant) or for too short a period of time (less than three weeks) and therefore do not respond to treatment.

13.3. Antidepressant drugs

The two major classes of antidepressants are tricyclic/tetracyclic antidepressants and monoamine oxidase inhibitors (MAOIs). Occasionally, stimulant drugs are also used to treat depressive states. Tryptophan and 5-hydroxy-tryptophan are also claimed to be useful.

13.4. Tricyclic/tetracyclic antidepressants and others

13.4.1. Classification

From a clinical point of view it is useful to subclassify tricyclic/tetracyclic antidepressant drugs in respect to their sedative effects.

13.4.2. Mild or nonsedative antidepressants

Imipramine, desipramine, nortriptyline, chlorimipramine, protriptyline, dibenzepine, lofepramine, carpipramine, nomifensin, trazodone.

13.4.3. Antidepressants with additional sedative actions

Amitriptyline, opipramol, doxepine, dothiepine, maprotiline, mianserine, butriptyline.

Action. When there is sedative action it precedes the antidepressant effects during the first week or two. The true antidepressant effect (against depressed mood, retardation, and apathy) has a delayed onset of two to four weeks (usually three). Antidepressant drugs with a so-called early onset of action are usually only quicker in sedation of the anxiety and tension but not in improvement of retardation or apathy. The sedative effect tends to diminish after a few days. Since three weeks is usually "par for the course," a shorter trial is inadequate to evaluate effectiveness.

Indications. Antidepressant drugs are indicated in all types of depressive states of different etiology (primary and secondary depression, reactive, neurotic, or so-called endogenous depressive states,

and depression secondary to physical or organic brain disorders).
The choice of the drug is dependent on the target syndrome (see
Part II).

Syndromes for which indicated

Primary
    4.1. Retarded depressive syndrome
    4.2. Agitated depressive syndrome
    4.3. Affective hypochondriacal syndrome
    4.4. Depressed obsessive-compulsive syndrome
    4.5. Depressive syndrome with delusions and hallucinations
    5.2. Phobic and obsessive-compulsive syndromes
    5.3. Depressive neurotic syndrome
    5.4. Neurotic hypochondriacal syndrome
    5.6. Neurasthenic syndrome
    6.5. Affective type of organic brain syndrome
    6.7. Post-traumatic cerebral syndromes
    6.8. Degenerative and demyelinating brain disorder syndromes
    7.1. Drug abuse syndrome
    7.2. Chronic alcoholic syndrome
    8.2. Enuresis nocturna syndrome
    8.3. Unmotivated retarded child syndrome

Secondary
    5.5. Hysterical syndrome
    5.5.1. Ganser's syndrome
    6.3. Cerebral arteriosclerotic syndrome
    6.4. Amnestic syndrome of senile dementia
    6.7. Post-traumatic cerebral syndromes
    8.1. Hyperkinetic syndrome (MBD, minimal brain dysfunction)

In combination with major tranquilizers
    2.1. Passive paranoid schizophrenic syndrome
    2.4. Catatonic schizophrenic syndrome
    2.7. Schizophrenic withdrawal syndrome

3.2. Depressive schizophrenic syndrome

4.7. Syndrome of simultaneous manic and depressive responses

5.7. Sexual neurotic syndrome

Caution. Pharmacologically the tricyclic/tetracyclic antidepressants are strong anticholinergic agents and should be used with caution in cardiovascular disease, liver disorders, epilepsy, glaucoma, urinary retention, pyloric stenosis, prostatic hypertrophy, and pregnancy. Use with caution in myocardial conduction disorders. Do not use for the first month after a myocardial infarct. Can aggravate narrow angle glaucoma (may increase intraocular tension). Not recommended if patient has history of thrombophlebitis.

Tolerance. Since tricyclic/tetracylic antidepressants are anticholinergic agents they provoke mainly autonomic side effects. Tricyclic/tetracyclic drugs can alter the pharmacological effect of other drugs administered concurrently, e.g., MAOIs, barbiturates, alcohol, methyldopa, guanethidine, and local anesthetics containing noradrenaline. There are claims that barbiturates may interfere with the action of these drugs through enzyme induction.

13.4.4. Side effects

The most common side effects of antidepressant drugs are tabulated below. Except for dryness of the mucosa, even the "common" side effects occur rather infrequently. There are small differences between different substances in respect to autonomic activity (anticholinergic action) and sedation. With rare exceptions the side effects tend to disappear with continuing treatment.

Sedation, weakness, fatigue, somnolence
Disturbance of visual accommodation
Dryness of the mucosa (mouth, nose, vagina)
Mydriasis
Sweating
Tachycardia, arrhythmia
EKG-changes (flattening of T-wave)

Hypotension (postural)
Constipation or diarrhea
Inhibition of micturition
Nausea, vomiting
Increase of body weight
Eosinophilia
Leukopenia, agranulocytosis
Change of erythrocyte sedimentation rate
Thromboses, thrombophlebitis
Jaundice, transitional changes of SGOT/SGPT, alkaline phosphatase
Allergic skin reactions, edema of the skin
Galactorhea, gynaecomastia, amenorrhea
Tremor
Epileptic seizures
Atonia of the intestine especially the ileum
Insomnia
Agitation, anxiety
Delirious states
Activation of schizophrenic symptoms

Resistance to treatment. In cases of resistance to a tricyclic/ tetracyclic one should always try another one; if this fails the next choice would be an MAO-inhibitor and following that a combination of both. But it is *not* advisable to first give an MAO-inhibitor and follow it several weeks later with full doses of a tricyclic or tetracyclic antidepressant, as dangerous collapse or rise of blood pressure may occur.

13.5. Monoamine oxidase inhibitors

Action. Chemically the MAO inhibitors can be subdivided into hydrazine and nonhydrazine derivatives; from a psychiatric point of view there is no difference in clinical action. Both types of MAOI inhibit the monoamine oxidase activity in mitochondria. Oral administration provides the greatest blockade of hepatic enzymes.

To achieve biochemical antidepressant action an 80 percent inhibition of MAOI in blood platelets is necessary (Nies et al. [156]).

More recent investigations have shown that there may exist heredi-
tary subtypes of MAOI-acetylators responding differently to the
MAOIs (Johnstone and Marsh [110]). There exist also subtypes A
and B of MAO inhibition (Youdim [240]), but up to now there is no
evidence of differential effects.

It is very important to know that despite the fact that MAOIs
themselves may be eliminated within twenty-four hours
(e.g.,tranylcypromine) or else within forty-eight hours, the enzyme-
inhibition may persist for one to two weeks. The consequence of
MAO-inhibition is an increase in brain serotonin level as well as in
norepinephrine and dopamine content in all tissue sites where these
amines are stored. Consequently, many other endogenous substances
may be altered in their metabolism, inducing unwanted side effects
such as tyramine potentiation. MAOIs can also have direct action
on excitability or transmission in the CNS (Valzelli [230]).

Initial clinical effect with MAOIs often requires twenty-one days
of treatment. Methods for selection of appropriate patients are under
investigation. Opinion ranges from the position that it is not possible
(Hamilton [86]) to the claim that suitable subjects can be selected
on the basis of rapidity of acetylation (Johnstone and Marsh [110]).

Tranylcypromine may have the quickest onset of action and is
also somewhat stimulant because it has an amphetamine-like side
chain.

Indications.   Depressive syndromes resistant to other drugs, atypical
depressions, phobic-compulsive anxiety states.

Combination with tricyclic/tetracyclic antidepressants.   After an initial treatment with an MAOI, subsequent treatment with large doses
of a tricyclic/tetracyclic antidepressant should be undertaken only
after a drug-free interval. There is a disagreement as to how long
this interval should be, with opinions ranging from a few days to
one to two weeks. The tricyclic should be started at a very low dose.
On the other hand, it is possible to combine both drugs, either
starting with a tricyclic/tetracyclic and adding an MAOI or starting
with both together. In this case additional caution is required: at
times the dosage of the tricyclic/tetracyclic antidepressant has to be
lowered by 50 percent and monitoring of blood pressure is necessary.
The combination of the two drugs should be restricted to skilled
psychopharmacologists (Shopsin and Kline 09].

Tricyclics/tetracyclics may be added to the regimen of a patient already on anMAOI. Since the tetracyclics release biogenic amines from their storage sites, this must be done very gradually: a sudden flood of such amines could lead to marked side effects.

Interaction with other drugs and food. MAOIs interact with many other substances, such as aminopyrine, acetanilide, cocaine, meperidine, and reserpine. Tricyclics/tetracyclics may be added to the regimen of a patient already on an MAOI. Since the tetracyclics release biogenic amines from their storage sites, this must be done very gradually: a sudden flood of such amines could lead to marked side effects. It is highly desirable to provide a patient with a printed set of instructions when an MAOI is prescribed. Except for very low doses of isocarboxazid (Marplan), it is desirable to have the patient adhere to certain restrictions of food, drink and medication. Care should be taken to explain that reactions to such substances are not always regular in occurrence. The fact that the patient deliberately or accidentally ingests a proscribed substance without ill-effects provides small assurance that a reaction may not occur the next time. Obviously, if the patient obtains no side effects to numerous items on the list provided, it will encourage disregard for the caution. Therefore it is actually dangerous to include on the list items that have not been clearly shown to be dangerous; the more substances included, the higher the probability of noncompliance.

The printed instructions provided by one of us (N.S.K.) follows. Based on extensive experience, a number of substances such as chocolate, bananas, etc. have not been included since evidence of their likelihood of producing side effects is isolated, tenuous, or based on unsubstantiated theoretical considerations. Obviously those responsible for the patient's diet should be alert for evidence that other items should be added.

INSTRUCTIONS TO PATIENTS ON MONAMINE OXIDASE INHIBITORS (MAOIs)

Patients on MAOIs (monamine oxidase inhibitors such as Eutonyl, Furoxone, Marplan, Nardil, and Parnate must beware of certain substances while on medication and for two weeks after stopping them.

Food

Do *not* eat cheeses except:	Cream and cottage cheese, yogurt and cheeses labeled "processed" (that is, in which fermentation has been stopped). One or two slices of ordinary pizza made with mozarella is safe.
Do *not* eat or drink stews or drinks made with meat extracts or yeast extracts	Meat itself (including stews) and natural gravies are safe. It is only gravies, drinks, or other products made from meat extracts that should be avoided. Bakery products made with yeast are allowed but not uncooked yeast.
Do *not* eat the following:	
Pickled herring;	Freshly prepared, frozen or tinned food is safe.
Chicken livers, goose livers and pate de foie gras;	
Food which has been aged without refrigeration (particularly meat and poultry);	
Broad bean pods (as served in some Chinese dishes)	
Do *not* take alcohol in more than small amounts	Limit yourself to three or four cans of beer.
Do *not* take sherry or red wines:	Limit yourself to two glasses (4 ounces each) of white wine or two glasses (1½ ounces each) of whisky, scotch, vodka, etc. Wine used in cooking is safe.
Avoid food or drink which has made you uncomfortable in the past or to which you know you are allergic.	

The literature on this subject occasionally refers to other foods. The evidence that these may cause trouble is not very certain. Therefore we have not listed them here. Several patients have inquired about bananas—these are perfectly safe. It is only the peel which contains large quantities of potentially dangerous material. Chocolate in reasonable amounts is also fine.

Medicines

Do *not* take any medications except:

Aspirin, Tylenol, Bufferin or antibiotics without consulting a doctor who knows you are on MAOIs. Vitamins and antibiotics are also safe, as are citrate or milk of magnesia and enemas. Medications such as Gelusil or metamucil used to reduce gastric acidity tend to interfere with absorption of other medications. They should not be taken at the same time but at least two hours apart.

Particularly Avoid:

Nasal decongestants such as Contac, as well as other preparations used for coughs and colds. If in doubt consult with your doctor or nurse.

Injections for dental work are safe if *Adrenalin* is *avoided* or *limited.*

If an operation is needed, MAOIs are usually discontinued a week or two in advance. In case of an emergency operation, be sure the surgeon anesthetist knows you are on an MAOI. Demerol should *not* be used for pain. Opium and morphine may be used as needed.

An unfavorable reaction usually produces a severe "pounding" headache caused by a marked rise in blood pressure. If this occurs go to the emergency room of a hospital rather than to a doctor's office.

Oral amphetamines and related substances in low doses are safe but they should *never* be given by injection.

An interaction is possible with indirectly acting sympathomimetic amines (parenteral amphetamine, fenfluramine, ephedrine, phenyl-propanolamine, tricyclic/tetracyclic antidepressants, barbiturates, hypnotics, pethidine and other narcotics, antihistamines, antihyper-tensives, hypoglycemics, insulin).

Syndromes for which indicated

Primary
- 4.1. Retarded depressive syndrome
- 4.3. Affective hypochondriacal syndrome
- 4.4. Depressed obsessive-compulsive syndrome
- 4.5. Depressive syndrome with delusions and hallucinations
- 5.2. Phobic and obsessive-compulsive syndrome
- 5.3. Depressive neurotic syndrome

Secondary
- 5.1. Anxiety state or syndrome
- 5.4. Neurotic hypochondriacal syndrome
- 8.5. Autistic child syndrome

In combination with major tranquilizers

- 2.1. Passive paranoid schizophrenic syndrome
- 2.4. Catatonic schizophrenic syndrome
- 2.7. Schizophrenic withdrawal syndrome
- 3.2. Depressive-schizophrenic syndrome
- 4.7. Syndrome of simultaneous manic and depressive responses
- 5.7. Sexual neurotic syndrome

Contraindications.   MAOIs are not absolutely contraindicated but should be used with caution in organic brain lesions, schizophrenic syndromes, epilepsy, pheochromocytoma, liver disease, cardiac decompensation, and congestive heart failure, and in combination with such incompatible drugs as are mentioned above.

Tolerance.   Tolerance of MAOIs is generally good. The main hazard is the incompatibility with many other substances, a drawback making MAOIs more difficult to handle than tricyclics/tetracyclics. Side effects are mainly autonomic (blood pressure, pulse rate, dizziness, and mental confusion have been reported).

Side effects.   The unwanted effects of MAOIs can be disturbing. The following list enumerates only the most important side effects:

Decrease of blood pressure, circulatory collapse
Sudden increase of blood pressure
Impotence, reduced sexual sensitivity, delayed orgasm
Headache
Insomnia (reduced need for sleep)
Toxic confusional states
Activation of schizophrenic syndromes
Epileptic seizures (reduced threshold)
Jaundice
Incompatibility with other drugs (see above)

13.6. Stimulants

Action. Psychostimulant drugs are characterized by an intense stimulation of certain brain structures with an ergotropic function. There may be brief initial sedation. Most of these drugs activate not only the central nervous system but also have peripheral functions including a peripheral sympathomimetic effect. Clinically these stimulants induce motor activity, hyperactivity in general, excitation, insomnia, inhibition of appetite, sometimes euphoria, and, at larger dosages, tremor and motor stereotypes.

Indications. Psychostimulant drugs are used for the treatment of narcolepsy, hyperkinetic syndromes of children (MBD), and occasionally of therapy-resistant depression with retarded or apathetic syndromes. Also of use in compensating for unwanted sedation induced by other drugs.

Syndromes for which indicated

Primary
    8.1. Hyperkinetic syndrome (minimal brain dysfunction)

Secondary
    4.1. Retarded depressive syndrome
    5.3. Depressive neurotic syndrome

Contraindications. Patients with schizophrenic syndromes treated with stimulant drugs may show marked deterioration. Stimulants should be avoided in individuals with a tendency to drug dependence.

Surprisingly, the risk of dependency is low when used in depressed patients.

Side effects.   In some patients there is development of tolerance and drug dependence. Long-term use at high doses may produce a condition clinically indistinguishable from paranoid schizophrenia. The following is a list of side effects:

> Tremor
> Tachycardia
> Hypertensive crisis
> Dryness of the mouth
> Anorexia, loss of body weight
> Impotence
> Insomnia
> Anxiety
> Hyperirritability, overstimulation
> Motor stereotypes
> Compulsive behavior
> Epileptic seizures
> Activation of schizophrenic symptoms

13. Antidepressants

Generic Name	Trade Name			Usual Dosage
	U.K.	U.S.	Canada	
Tricyclic Antidepressants				
Amitriptyline (156)	Tryptizol Saroten Lentizol Domical Amizol	Elavil SK-amitriptylene Endep Amitril	Elavil Meravil Novotriptyn Amilene Deprex Levate	75–300 mg
Trimepramine (245)	Surmontil		Surmontil	50–100 mg
Opipramol (227)	Insidon			150–300 mg
Doxepin (187)	Sinequan	Sinequan Adapin	Sinequan	30–300 mg
Imipramine (206)	Tofranil Berkomine Co-caps Imipramine Demipressin Norpramine Oppanyl Praminil	Tofranil Antipress Imavate Janimine Presamine SK-pramine	Tofranil Impril Novopramine Praminil	o: 75–150 mg i: 75–300 mg
Chlorimipramine (165) (clomipramine)	Anafranil			75–300 mg
Nortriptyline (223)	Aventyl Allegron	Aventyl Pamelar	Aventyl	75–300 mg
Desipramine (182)	Pertofran	Pertofrane Norpramin	Pertofrane Norpramin	75–300 mg
Dibenzepin (184)	Noveril			240–620 mg
Clofepramine (171) (Trade Name: Lopramine)				90–210 mg

Generic Name	Trade Name			Usual Dosage
	U.K.	U.S.	Canada	
Carpipramine (164)				150–300 mg
Butriptyline (162)	Evadyne			75–150 mg
Protriptyline (236)	Concordin-s	Vivactil	Triptil	10–80 mg
Prothiaden (235) (Dothiepin)	Prothiaden			75–150 mg
Tetracyclic Antidepressants				
Maprotiline (1252)	Ludiomil	Ludiomil	Ludiomil	75–150 mg
Mianserine				10–40 mg
Other structures				
Tofenacine (1259)	Elamol			240 mg
Iprindol (397)	Prondol			45–120 mg
Trazodone (994)				75–150 mg
Nomifensin				
L-tryptophan combined with pyridoxin and ascorbic acid	Optimax			12 tablets daily
Combinations				
Amitriptyline (156)	Triptafen-DA	Etrafon	Etrafon	
Perphenazine(86)	Triptafen-Forte	Triavil	Triavil	
	Triptafen-Minor			
Amitriptyline (156)	Limbitrol	Limbitrol		
Chlordiazepoxide (523)				
Fluphenazine Dihydrochloride (47)	Motival			
Nortriptyline (223)				

Generic Name	Trade Name			Usual Dosage
	U.K.	U.S.	Canada	
Monoamine oxidase inhibitors				
Iproniazid (776)	Marsilid			75–150 mg daily
Isocarboxazide (777)	Marplan / Isocarboxazid	Marplan	Marplan	30–90 mg daily
Nialamide (867)	Niamid	Withdrawn from Market		75–300 mg daily
Pargyline (1370)	Eutonyl	Eutonyl		10–200 mg daily
Phenelzine (1165)	Nardil	Nardil	Nardil	45–90 mg daily
Tranylcypromine (1192)	Parnate	Parnate	Parnate	30–80 mg daily
Combination				
Tranylcypromine (1192) 10 mg / Trifluoperazine (130) 1 mg	Parstelin			3–15 mg daily
Stimulants				
Dextroamphetamine (1098)	Dexedrine / Dexamed	Dexedrine	Dexedrine	*o: 5–30 mg / *i:30–60 mg
Methamphetamine (1147)		Desoxyn		o: 2.5–15 mg / i: 15–30 mg
Methylphenidate	Ritalin	Ritalin	Ritalin / Methidate	o: 10–30 mg / i: 30–60 mg
Piperadrol (931)				o: 2– 4 mg / i: 4–10 mg

Generic Name	Trade Name			Usual Dosage
	U.K.	U.S.	Canada	
Combinations				
Methamphetamine (1147) Amobarbital (563)		Adipex Ty-med		
Methamphetamine (1147) Phenobarbital-Na		Desbutal		
Dextroamphetamine (1098) Amobarbital (563)		Dexamyl		
Dextroamphetamine (1098) Prochlorperazine (95)		Eskatrol		

*o = outpatient / *i = inpatient

14. MINOR TRANQUILIZERS

14.1. Definition of anxiety

Anxiety states or syndromes are characterized by inner anxiety, fear or panic, psychic and motor restlessness, loss of concentration, interference with capacity to enjoy (in contrast to loss of the capacity as in depression), and concomitant physical symptoms such as dryness of the mouth, constipation or diarrhea, tachycardia, mydriasis, and sweating. Most frequently anxiety is one of the symptoms of neurosis, alcoholism, psychosomatic disorders, and depression.

14.2. Principles of use

The drug treatment of anxiety is purely symptomatic. The available drugs can be classified into different groups, the preferred one being the group of dibenzodiazepines. They have a rather specific anxiolytic effect. Their toxicity is very low, and they are well tolerated, although some patients can develop tolerance or dependence. The dosage has to be adapted individually.

14.3. Psychopharmacological treatment

Anxiety syndromes are best treated by minor tranquilizers of the group of dibenzodiazepines. There is a spectrum of different dibenzodiazepines available; at the one end are those with very weak, on the other end those with rather strong sedative effects. They are listed here, beginning with the less sedative and progressing to the more sedative. Tolerance is very high (see side effects below)

Lorazepam (Ativan). Dosage: 2–7.5 mg
Oxazepam (Serax, Serenid-D). Dosage: 15–150 mg
Chlordiazepoxide (Librium). Dosage: 20–100 mg (or higher)
Medazepam (Nobrium). Dosage: 15–60 mg
Diazepam (Valium). Dosage: 3–60 mg

Anxiety can also be treated by low dosages of the sedative major tranquilizers. These are particularly useful for patients who tend to be addiction-prone and in general for patients who require prolonged therapy. In patients who develop a tolerance or in those who develop marked dependence, the possibility of tardive dyskinesia from low doses of the sedative major tranquilizers seems the lesser of the disadvantages.

Action.   Minor tranquilizers are also called antianxiety or anxiolytic drugs. Another name is "ataraktika," derived from the Greek word *ataraktos* (undisturbed, intrepid), a state of mental balance described by the philosophical school of the Stoics. The term *tranquilizer* is derived from the Latin *tranquillitas*, meaning calmness of the wind or sea (167).

Pharmacologically, minor tranquilizers, in contrast to major tranquilizers, have no anti-psychotic and no extrapyramidal activity. There is either a very mild effect on autonomic nervous functions or none at all. Most minor tranquilizers inhibit polysynaptic reflexes of the spinal cord and at higher dosages inhibit conditioned reflexes. They therefore induce muscle relaxation. They are all more or less anticonvulsive. This special psychotropic effect is due to effects on deeper regions of the brain associated with emotion (limbic system, hypothalamus, and reticular system of the brain stem). An antianxiety agent is a substance which relieves anxiety and produces calmness, peacefulness, serenity, placidity or ataraxia. The term *antianxiety drug* does not mean that every symptom of anxiety can be counteracted, but it does mean that the effect is not restricted to specific diagnostic subtypes of mental disorders.

Minor tranquilizers have been widely used in the treatment of anxiety of various etiology. They have even been abused when taken for the "treatment" of the anxiety which occurs within normal life experience. They have also been abused by physicians who seek to relieve tension and anxiety in patients suffering from undiagnosed illnesses. Sometimes it is easier to prescribe a tranquilizer than to devote more time to a thorough examination of the patient.

Prescribing an antianxiety drug may mean that the doctor has decided to pursue a symptomatic target, symptom-oriented therapy neglecting etiology and pathogenesis. These minor tranquilizers do have a precise use which entails a precise psychiatric diagnosis. It is really necessary before prescribing such a drug to be certain that it is not being used out of ignorance to replace psychotherapy or some other type of medication (antidepressant, major tranquilizer) which is really indicated.

Indications. The indications for antianxiety drugs are therefore very broad since they may be used in combination with other types of therapy or other drugs. It is impossible to enumerate all the physical and mental disorders that may induce a primary or secondary anxiety syndrome. Antianxiety drugs have been used to tranquilize patients before surgical and obstetrical procedures; to relieve tension and anxiety in the treatment of many psychosomatic disorders; to break vicious circles; and to treat gastrointestinal disturbances, allergies, dermatitis, and headaches. Pain can be influenced not only by the psychotropic effect but also by the muscle relaxant properties of these drugs (rheumatology). Minor tranquilizers are also useful in the treatment of early insomnia, in inducing relief from tension, and in decreasing concern about emotional problems. They are useful as adjuvants in the treatment of the agitated depressive syndrome. In such severe psychotic states as the schizophrenic syndromes, the major tranquilizers are obviously indicated. Minor tranquilizers, however, may be useful for the sedation of severe brain disorder syndromes (e.g., delirium tremens, arteriosclerotic confusion), but special caution in these cases is indicated because elderly patients and those with brain damage may be particularly sensitive to drugs. On the other hand, children have been widely treated with minor tranquilizers in low dosages with good effect; of course, one has to remember in this respect that learning may possibly be impaired by habitual use of psychotropic drugs.

Syndromes for which indicated

Primary
- **5.1.** Anxiety state or syndrome
- **5.4.** Neurotic hypochondriacal syndrome
- **5.5.** Hysterical syndrome
- **5.5.1.** Ganser's syndrome
- **6.6.1.1.** Petit-mal syndrome (diazepam, intravenously)
- **6.6.4.** Character disorder syndromes of epileptic origin
- **6.7.** Post-traumatic cerebral syndromes
- **7.1.** Drug abuse syndrome
- **7.3.** Alcohol-induced delirium syndrome
- **7.5.** Withdrawal syndromes
- **9.** Oligophrenic syndrome

Secondary
- **4.2.** Agitated depressive syndrome
- **4.3.** Affective hypochondriacal syndrome
- **5.2.** Phobic and obsessive-compulsive syndromes
- **5.3.** Depressive neurotic syndrome
- **5.6.** Neurasthenic syndrome
- **5.7.** Sexual neurotic syndrome
- **6.3.** Cerebral arteriosclerotic syndrome
- **6.5.** Affective type of organic brain syndrome
- **6.7.** Post-traumatic cerebral syndromes
- **7.2.** Chronic alcoholic syndrome
- **8.1.** Hyperkinetic syndrome (minimal brain dysfunction)
- **8.4.** Syndrome of periodic episodes of disturbed behavior

In any condition in which anxiety is not controlled by the major type of therapy.

Tolerance. The main side effects of minor tranquilizers are over-sedation, muscle relaxation (sudden falling in elderly people), and drowsiness. Prolonged use carries a risk of dependence. This is especially true for meprobamate. The benzodiazepines taken in excessive dosages also can create a drug dependence in subjects prone to addiction.

Abrupt withdrawal symptoms from high doses include seizures. The toxicity of minor tranquilizers in general is rather low, the rare suicide resulting mainly from meprobamate. The toxic state is similar to barbiturate intoxication (coma) except that flaccid muscles lead to a more marked drop in blood pressure. If fluids are given in quantity to support the blood pressure there is a real danger, when muscle tonus returns, of overburdening the cardiovascular system with excess fluid. Phlebotomy may be necessary in severe cases.

Side effects.   Minor tranquilizers are doubtlessly the best tolerated psychotropic drugs. This is especially true for the group of benzodiazepines. They are so well tolerated that it may be difficult to develop better drugs for the treatment of anxiety states. The drugs on the market have very much in common. Differences exist mainly in the sedative effects. The following is a list of side effects:

> Oversedation, somnolence
> Dizziness, ataxia
> Muscle relaxation
> Loss of libido, impotence
> Confusion
> Agitation, hostility
> Hypotension
> Weight increase
> Vertigo
> Drowsiness
> Lowered tolerance for alcohol
> Skin reactions
> Drug dependence
> Disarthria
> Paradoxical effects (stimulation)
> Increased muscular tension
> Breathlessness
> Choking
> Palpitations
> Trembling
> Insomnia

14. Minor tranquilizers

Generic Name	Trade Name			Usual Dosage
	U.K.	U.S.	Canada	
Dibenzodiazepine derivatives				
Chlorazepate (522)	Tranxene	Tranxene	Tranxene	15–60 mg (only for adults and teenagers over 12 years)
Chlordiazepoxide (523)	Librium Calmoden Tropium	Librium Libritabs A-poxide	Librium Medilium Nack Novopoxide Protensin Relaxil Solium Trilium	20–100 mg children: 5–20 mg
Diazepam (528)	Valium Atensine Tensium	Valium	Valium D-tran E-pam Erital Meval Novodipam Paxel Neo-calme Serenack Stress Pam Vivol	5–60 mg
Lorazepam (533)	Ativan Nobrium	Ativan	Ativan	2–7.5 mg
Medazepam (534)				10–60 mg
Oxazepam (538)	Serenid-D Serenid Forte	Serax	Serax	15–150 mg

Generic Name	Trade Name			Usual Dosage
	U.K.	U.S.	Canada	
Other chemical structures				
Meprobamate (1446)	Equanil	Equanil	Equanil	400–1200 mg
	Mepavlon	Meprobamate	Quital	children:
	Meprate	Meprospan	Landol	200–400 mg
	Milonorm	Meprotabs	Meditran	
	Miltown	Meprotil	Mep-E	
	Tenavoid	Miltown	Meprospan	
	Tised		Miltown	
			Neo-tran	
			Novomepro	
Hydroxyzine (768)	Atarax	Atarax	Atarax	50–100 mg
Hydroxyzine pamoate	Equipose	Vistaril		75–400 mg
Methylpentynol (1470)	Oblivon			500–1000 mg
	Insomnol			
Methylpentynol carbamate (1447)	Oblivon-C			100–200 mg
Benzoctamine (1104)	Tacitin			10–60 mg
Chlormethazanone (704)	Trancopal	Trancopal	Trancopal	200–600 mg

Generic Name	Trade Name			Usual Dosage
	U.K.	U.S.	Canada	
Prothipendyl (938)	Tolnate			40–120 mg
Methocarbamol (1361)	Robaxin Robaxintate	Robaxin	Robaxin	500–4000 mg
Tybamate (1451)		Tybatran		250–2000 mg
Benactyzine (1212)				40–200 mg
Phenaglycodol (1371)				300–1200 mg
Captodiame (1242)		Suvren		100–400 mg
Diphenhydramine (1244)	Benadryl	Benadryl SK-diphenhydramine	Benadryl	25–50 mg
Combinations	Amorgyl			3 × 1
	Amylozine			1 – 3
	Bellergal			3 × 1 – 2
	Drinamyl			1 – 3
	Elixier Gabail			3 × 10 ml
	Halabar			3 – 6
	Passiorine			3 × 5 – 10 ml
	Tenavoid	Baucaps		3 × 1
		Librax		3 × 1
		Medigesic		3 × 1

15. HYPNOTICS

Action. Hypnotics are rapidly absorbed and either quickly or slowly eliminated; complete elimination takes from a few hours to several days. Most of these drugs suppress REM-sleep and after withdrawal there is an increase of REM-time for days or weeks. Barbiturates stimulate microsomal enzymes and therefore accelerate not only their own metabolism but also the metabolism of other drugs, e.g., the tricyclic/tetracyclic antidepressants. This increased catabolism therefore may diminish the effectiveness of the tricyclics/ tetracyclics.

The depressive effect spreads over the entire central nervous system, especially the cerebral cortical areas. High dosages induce somnolence and coma. Barbiturates are strong anticonvulsant agents and the effect is potentiated by most of the major tranquilizers. Hypnotics have a depressant effect on the cardiovascular, respiratory, and gastrointestinal systems. In low dosages their effect is sedative, in high dosages hypnotic. Barbiturates can be subclassified in respect to their duration of action into three groups; short-acting, medium-acting, and long-acting compounds. The short-acting barbiturates are amobarbital, hexobarbital, secobarbital, and thiopental; medium action is produced by aprobarbital, butabarbital, cyclobarbital, and heptabarbital; and a long-lasting effect results from phenobarbital. The action can be intensified and prolonged by the administration of a potentiating sedative major tranquilizer, for instance, methotrimeprazine, clozapine, or chlorpromazine. Hypnotics with a long-lasting effect tend to accumulate, and some patients may therefore suffer from hypnotic hangover in the morning.

Indications.   Hypnotics are indicated only after failure of minor tranquilizers or sedative major tranquilizers. Nonbarbiturate hypnotics are preferable to barbiturates. However, barbiturates may be especially indicated in late insomnia (early wakening in the morning) such as occurs in depression.

Barbiturates are too frequently given for the treatment of insomnia, and in all cases one must be aware of the danger of drug dependence. Some barbiturates (amobarbital, thiopental) are given intravenously for narcoanalysis.

Contraindications.   Coma, porphyria (barbiturates).

Relative contraindications.   Liver damage, renal insufficiency, myasthenia gravis. An unpredictable interaction with alcohol can be dangerous. The hypnotic effect may then be less than the repression of respiration which creates a real danger. There also tends to be cross tolerance with alcohol. Barbiturates are found in the milk of the lactating mother so that, if possible, they should not be given during pregnancy or the period of lactation.

Withdrawal.   The withdrawal syndromes of barbiturate and other hypnotic dependency include insomnia, weakness, tremor, anxiety, delirium (similar to delirium tremens), and epileptic seizures. The withdrawal symptoms can be prevented by slow decrease of the dosage alone or in combination with the administration of clomethiazole.

15. Hypnotics

Generic Name	Trade Name U.K.	Trade Name U.S.	Trade Name Canada	Usual Dosage
Barbiturates				
*m Aprobarbital (564)		Alurate		40 mg
s Amobarbital (563)	Amylomet Amytal	Amytal	Amytal Isosec	100 –200 mg
Amobarbital-Na	Sodium Amytal	Amytal Sodium		
m Butabarbital (566)	Soneryl	Buticaps Butisol Sodium	Butibard Butisol Daybarb Neobarb	100–200 mg
m Cyclobarbital (570)	Phanodorm Rapidal			
m Heptabarbital (574)	Medomin		Medomin	200 –400 mg
Pentobarbital (583)		Nembutal Sodium	Novo Rectal Nembutal Pentogen	30–50 mg
Mephobarbital (578)	Prominal	Mebaral		
l Phenobarbital (584)	Gardenal Phenobarbitone Luminal	SK-phenobarbitol	Eskabarb Gardenal Luminal Novo-pheno	60–100 mg
s Secobarbital (586)	Seconal Sodium	Seconal Seconal Sodium	Secogen Seconal Seral	
s Thiopental (589)	Interval	Pentothal	Pentothal	
s Hexobarbital (576)	Hexobarbitone	Sombulex		260–520 mg

* s = short acting   m = medium acting   l = long acting

Generic Name	Trade Name				Usual Dosage
	U.K.	U.S.	Canada		
Non-Barbiturates					
Chloral Hydrate (1413)		Aquachloral	Chloralex		1000–2000 mg
		Noctec	Chloralven		
		SK-chloral hydrate	Noctec		
			Novochlorhydrate		
Chlorhexadol	Medodorm				350–370 mg
Clomethiazole (708)	Heminevrin				500 mg
Dichloralphenazone	Welldorm		Chloralol		1– 2 g
Ethchlorvynol (1465)	Serenesil	Placidyl	Placidyl		500 mg
Ethinamate (1442)		Valmid	Valmid		up to 1 g
Flurazepam (530)	Dalmane	Dalmane	Dalmane		15–60 mg
Glutethimide (758)	Doriden	Doriden	Doriden		250 –1000 mg
Methylpentynol Carbamate (1447)	Insomnol				350–700 mg (children less)
	Oblivon				
Methyprylon (849)	Noludar	Noludar	Noludar		200–400 mg
Methaqualon (843)	Revonal	Parest	Mequelon		200–400 mg
		Quaalude	Methadorm		
		Sopor	Rouqualone		
			Sedalone		
			Triadone		
			Tualone		
			Vitalone		
Nitrazepam (536)	Mogadon				5–10 mg
	Remnos				

16. OTHER DRUGS

16.1. Carbamazepine (163) - Tegretol (U.K.), Tegretal

Action. Mood stabilizing, activating (in epilepsy). Increases activity, interest, learning abilities, and contact in epileptic children. Anticonvulsive, analgesic (trigeminal neuralgia), antiarrhythmic.

Indications. Disturbances of mood and behavior in epileptic patients (aggressive, suspicious, intolerant, subject to apparently irrational outbursts). Especially indicated in localized focal seizures (particularly psychomotor seizures). In most of cases it should be combined with Phenytoin. Second choice for behavior disturbances in oligophrenia and TLE (temporal lobe epilepsy) in children of normal intelligence.

Contraindication. Use with caution in combination with MAOIs.

Syndromes for which indicated

Primary
   6.6.1.2. Temporal lobe seizure syndrome (psychomotor attacks)
   6.6.2.1. After psychomotor attacks
      6.6.4. Character disorder syndromes of epileptic origin
         6.7. Post-traumatic cerebral syndromes

Secondary
   8.3. Unmotivated retarded child syndrome
   8.4. Syndrome of periodic episodes of disturbed behavior

Effect on EEG: Increase in abnormality, increase in paroxysmal abnormalities may occur.

Dosage: Initially 100–200, increase until 800–1200 mg. In children: 7.3–30.5 mg/Kg.

16.2. Lithium

Lithium was introduced into psychiatry by the Australian Cade [43], who in 1949 reported having detected its sedative effect on animals. He then applied it to the manic syndromes. It was first recommended as a therapeutic agent for acute and later for chronic hypomanic syndromes. It does not act rapidly, so it cannot compete with *major tranquilizers* in the very acute conditions; it can, however, be combined with them in a very effective manner. Lithium may also have some antidepressant effect, noted first by Voijtechovsky in 1957 (231), but it cannot compete with the modern antidepressives.

The detection of a prophylactic action of lithium against recurrent affective disorders was a milestone in the history of modern psychiatry. The first reports by Hartigan (91) and Baastrup (23) were based on independent clinical observations. Subsequently Mogens Schou (194–199) devoted his full work to the question of the prophylactic effect of lithium on manic depressive disorders and together with Baastrup (23) carried out the first systematic study based on an intraindividual comparison of two periods of observation (without treatment, under treatment). The critical objections of Blackwell and Shepherd (34), Lader (127), and Saran (192) in England were disproved a few years later by the application of other methods, using multiple regression analysis (Angst and Weis [11]) and double-blind trials (22, 47, 49, 106, 147, 170, 173, 220).

Today the prophylactic action of lithium is well established, proven not only by double-blind trials but also by a study of cessation of treatment after a few years (Baastrup et al. [22]), which showed relapse of patients on placebo but not of those on lithium.

Action.   Lithium reduces amplitude and duration of affective episodes, prolongs the free interval, or extinguishes completely the
entire course of cyclic episodes.

Indications.   Lithium salts are indicated, first of all, as long-term
prophylactic treatment against recurrent bipolar manic-depressive
disorders, recurrent depression, and recurrent mania. It can also be
used against recurrent schizoaffective disorders (Angst et al. [7]) as
well as depressive syndromes of mixed neurotic-endogenous etiology.
It has been tried in recurrent schizophrenic syndromes mainly of the
catatonic type, but here the effect is not established.

Preparations.   Lithium salts are available in different forms of
varying molecular weight. The standard unit for dosage is measured
by 1 milliequivalent (meq) = 1 mval = 1 mmol = 6.9 mg lithium.
This amount is equivalent to

> 66 mg Li-acetate
> 154 mg Li-adipate
> 37 mg Li-carbonate
> 94 mg Li-citrate
> 200 mg Li-gluconate
> 154 mg Li-glutamate
> 55 mg Li-sulfate

Because of its worldwide use it is important to be able to compare
the different preparations. The following are on the market:

> Lithium carbonicum, 250 mg carbonate
> = 6.8 meq Li
> Quilonum, 536 mg acetate
> = 8.1 meq Li
> Quilonum retard, 450 mg carbonate
> = 12.2 meq Li
> Lithionit Duretter and Lithium Duriles, 330 mg sulfate
> = 6.0 meq
> Hypnorex, 400 mg carbonate
> = 10.8 meq Li

Lithiofor, 660 mg sulfate
$$= 12.0 \text{ meq Li}$$

U.S.:   Eskalith, 300 mg carbonate
Lithane, 300 mg carbonate
Lithium carbonate, 300 mg carbonate
Lithonate, 300 mg carbonate

U.K.:   Camcolit, 250 mg carbonate
$$= 6.8 \text{ meq Li}$$
Lithium Phasal, 300 mg carbonate
Priadel (sustained release), 400 mg carbonate
$$= 10.8 \text{ meq Li}$$

Dosage.   Lithium prophylaxis is usually started slowly, the therapeutic dose being built up within about two weeks. It is recommended that treatment begin with 1/2–1 tablet per day and that this
dosage be increased every three days until the blood concentration
for prophylactic effect is reached. In physically normal young or
middle-aged adults this usually should be between 0.5 and 1.2
meq/1. The blood sample should be taken ten hours ± two hours
after the last dose. The absorption of lithium is very rapid and the
peak in the blood level is reached after about two hours. For this
reason some clinicians prefer sustained-release tablets, though others
do not consider the serum level so important but are more concerned
with the total daily dose. In some cases, particularly elderly individuals, blood levels of 0.3 and 0.4 are adequate. Dose varies considerably due to differences in absorption, retention, and excretion. For
the treatment of manic syndromes, higher dosages may be necessary,
with blood concentrations of about 1.7 meq/1. For prophylactic
treatment the average dose is 3 × 300 mg lithium carbonate or 2
× 1 or 2 tablets of a sustained released form.

Contraindications.   Insufficient renal clearance, conditions disturbing sodium balance, severe cardiac disease. Sodium-free diet as
indicated.

Caution.   Pregnancy, hypothyroidism.

Syndromes for which indicated

Primary (prophylaxis of)
3.1. Manic-schizophrenic syndrome
4.1. Retarded depressive syndrome
4.2. Agitated depressive syndrome
4.3. Affective hypochondriacal syndrome
4.5. Depressive syndrome with delusions and hallucinations
4.6. Manic-hypomanic syndrome
4.7. Syndrome of simultaneous manic and depressive responses

Secondary
5.3. Depressive neurotic syndrome
5.4. Neurotic hypochondriacal syndrome
10. Endocrine psychosyndrome (premenstrual tension)

Tolerance. Initial side effects: gastrointestinal (nausea, vomiting, diarrhea), tremor.

Late side effects. Tremor, increase of body weight, exacerbation of acne, euthyroid struma, polyuria, polydipsia, reversible renal diabetes insipidus.

Treatment of side effects. Propanolol (2 × 40 mg) against lithium tremor, antithyroid medication against euthyroid struma or thyroid replacements for hypofunction of thyroid. Digitalis in cases of impending cardiac decompensation due to the increased turnover of water.

16.3. Antiparkinson drugs

Action. Anticholinergic, antiparkinson effect.

Indication. Antiparkinson drugs should be given only in cases of extrapyramidal symptoms or preventively in cases of oversensitivity to major tranquilizers. Patients on long-term major tranquilizers are frequently overtreated with antiparkinson drugs.

Tolerance.   Antiparkinson drugs are strong anticholinergic agents, creating such side effects as dryness of the mucosa, mydriasis, constipation, difficulty of micturation, tachycardia, delirious states, and mental confusion (especially when combined with anticholinergic major tranquilizers).

Relative contraindication.   Glaucoma, prostatic hypertrophy.

Not recommended.   L-Dopa is not effective in drug-induced parkinson syndromes.

16.3 Antiparkinson drugs

Generic Name	Trade Name			Usual Dosage
	U.K.	U.S.	Canada	
Benepryzine (1213)	Brizin			p.o. 50–200 mg
Benztropine (689)	Cogentin	Cogentin	Cogentin Bensylate	p.o. 1–4 mg i.m. 1–2 mg
Biperiden (690)	Akineton	Akineton	Akineton	p.o. 2–6 mg i.v. slowly or i.m. 5–20 mg daily
Chlorphenoxamine	Clorevan	Phenoxene	Phenoxene	p.o. 50–150 mg
Cycrimine (716)		Pagitane	Pargitane	1.25–5 mg
Diphenhydramin (1244)	Benadryl	Benadryl	Benadryl	p.o.25–50 mg
Profenamine (96) (Ethopropazine)			Parsitane	p.o.50–500 mg
Orphenadrine (1254)	Disipal	Disipal	Disipal Norflex	p.o. 150–400 mg i.m. 20–40 mg
Procyclidine (935)	Kemadrin	Kemadrin	Kemadrin	p.o. 7.5–60 mg
Trihexyphenidyl (995)	Artane, Trinol Artane sustets	Artane Tremin	Artane Aparkane Novohexidyl Trixyl	p.o. 2–10 mg p.o. 2–10 mg

Part IV. Side Effects

17. CARDIOVASCULAR

17.1. Blood pressure

17.1.1. Decrease in blood pressure

A decrease of blood pressure is frequently found in patients on psychopharmaceuticals, especially at the beginning of treatment. The most common type is postural hypotension. Antidepressant drugs are capable of reinforcing adrenergic mechanisms when administered in moderate doses, but when employed in high doses they may exert an antiadrenergic effect producing a drop in blood pressure. The hypotensive effect is stronger in phenothiazine derivatives with aliphatic sidechains and in piperidine groups than in phenothiazines with piperazinylalcyl side chains. The hypertensive patient in whom blood pressure is already labile (especially schizophrenics) (32) and elderly subjects are particularly susceptible to decreases in blood pressure. Not only the systolic pressure but especially the diastolic pressure can be lowered (58). The effect of long-term administration of psychotropic drugs is less well known but there is also frequently a small decrease of blood pressure to be found. Decrease of blood pressure induced by psychotropic drugs is important considering, for instance, that 5 percent of the population of Canada suffers cardiac disorders and that 50 percent of all deaths are of cardiovascular origin (24,25). Postural hypotension is observed mainly during the first days of treatment. The best technique of management is to have the patient lie down. If the hypotension persists, an elastic abdominal belt of the type used after hernia operations may be sufficient. Noradrenaline (norepinephrine) is not recommended because, contrary to what might be expected, this can result in blood pressure being decreased still further. A countereffect to the hypotension is exerted by dihydergot (DHE) and heptaminol. The true mechanism of the decrease of blood pressure has not been fully clarified. Vasodilatation has been found in animals but it is by no means certain that the same effect is produced in humans. The vasodilatation probably results from a direct effect of the drug on the arteries or via some central mechanism. Plethysmographic studies after brachial arterial injections of small amounts of chlorpromazine showed an increased blood flow to the hand.

When starting ambulatory treatment with a psychotropic drug it is frequently desirable during the first two or three days to give the drug only at night, in order to reduce the likelihood of hypotension. The subjective symptoms of hypotension experienced by the patient are reported to bear little correlation with the extent of the drop in blood pressure (42). Postural hypotension at times can be severe enough to induce collapse. Sudden drop of blood pressure has been observed mainly in patients with preexisting cardiovascular disorders, in elderly patients, and in combination treatment with MAO-inhibitors and drugs with adrenergic mechanisms; this results in a paradoxical decrease of blood pressure. Therefore, one should not combine MAO-inhibitors with adrenergic substances, and at least in theory (but not so much in practice) there is also an increased risk of blood pressure drop if an MAO-inhibitor is combined with a tricyclic antidepressant.

17.1.2. Increase in blood pressure

Increase in blood pressure induced by psychotropic drugs is rare, although it has been described in geriatric patients (26, 41, 143). A sudden increase of blood pressure also has been reported when tricyclic antidepressants were used subsequent to treatment with MAO-inhibitors. It seems to be less dangerous to give a simultaneous combination of the two types of drugs or to start with a tricyclic antidepressant and during this treatment to gradually add an MAO-inhibitor.

Reputed incompatibility between MAOIs and tricyclic antidepressants was first mentioned by Harrer (89, 90), who reported on a few patients who showed toxic effects including dizziness, nausea, vomiting, coarse tremor, headache, profuse sweating, dyspnoea, and collapse, as well as, in certain cases, delirium and confusion. Studies by Marks (142) revealed the importance of tyramine in the pathogenesis. The most frequent side effect is sharp decrease of blood pressure, but one occasionally finds an increase. Since these are the same side effects as would result from MAOIs alone, it is unclear whether the combination increases the probability of side effects.

In an extensive study Shopsin and Kline (209) reported on over 500 patients treated with MAOI-tricyclic combinations. The incidence of side effects was no greater than for either drug alone and there were no fatalities.

Parenterally administered adrenergic drugs are strongly contraindicated. They produce sweating, motor restlessness, hyperexcitability, hyperreflexia, clonus, Babinski sign, tremor, rigidity, opisthotonos, myoclonia, epileptic seizures, and progressive clouding of consciousness sometimes leading to coma. The blood pressure may drop sharply, the pulse increase, and marked hyperthermia develop with possibly fatal outcome. Orally administered, the adrenergic preparations seem relatively safe at ordinary doses.

17.2. Cardiac effects

Cardiotoxic effects of psychotropic drugs have been of increasing interest during the last few years. Clinical investigations have shown that long-term treatment in patients over fifty years of age can induce a definite effect on glycosides, leading at times to insufficiency of the heart as evaluated by experiments on performance. It is therefore recommended that in long-term treatment the physician look carefully for early symptoms of cardiac insufficiency and add, if necessary, digoxin or digitoxin.

The decrease of blood pressure is frequently associated with an increase in pulse rate. Some preparations (for instance, clozapine) may at times induce a rather marked tachycardia.

Electrocardiographic changes are produced mainly by tricyclic psychotropic drugs such as thioridazine or the tricyclic antidepressants. The most frequent changes are flattening or extension of T-waves or isoelectric or negative waves. Occasionally one can find a prolongation of P-R or Q-R interval or lowering of S-T and changes of the U-wave. These shifts of repolarization are not dangerous;

they seem to be unspecific and their importance overestimated. They can be seen quite frequently and are without any clinical relevance, although sometimes one can find disturbances of rhythm or extrasystoles. A quantitative relationship between dosage of drugs and T-waves has not been established (236). Disturbances of repolarization due to thioridazine can be normalized by the administration of ergotamine tartrate, isorbiddinitrate, and potassium. At the present time there is nothing known about pathological anatomic changes of the myocardium induced by psychotropic drugs (183).

The changes of rhythm or increase of heart rate can create palpitations such as has been observed under imipramine or clozapine.

18. AUTONOMIC

Psychotropic drugs frequently affect both adrenergic and cholinergic systems. Most of the tricyclic antidepressants as well as the phenothiazines are both adrenergic and anticholinergic, whereas the MAO-inhibitors are purely adrenergic. Autonomic side effects are generally mild and tend to diminish after one or two weeks. It is therefore recommended that the dosage be built up step by step, especially during the first three days, in order to give some time for adaptation.

18.1. Dryness of the mucosa

18.1.1. Dry mouth

Many patients suffer from a dry mouth as a consequence of anxiety and tension (especially in depression) and these symptoms may be increased by an antidepressant drug. Interestingly, the same effect can also be a consequence of placebo effect. Dryness of the oral mucosa may lead to glossitis, stomatitis, mouth ulcers, xerostomia, or even to secondary damage to the teeth. All these complications, however, are extremely rare. Objective measurement has shown that the secretion of saliva diminishes markedly. On the other hand, secretion of saliva may be one of the signs of autonomic nervous function which may possibly serve as an indicator of the patient's responsiveness to therapy (105a).

18.1.2. Dryness of the nasal mucosa

This dryness can induce constriction of breathing.

18.1.3. Dryness of the vagina

Dryness of the vagina has also been reported and can on rare occasions induce temporary frigidity.

18.2. Hypersalivation

Many antipsychotic drugs can induce hypersalivation as part of the parkinsonian syndrome. This can reach excessive amounts but usually responds to treatment with an antiparkinsonian drug. Clozapine, an agent that does not create a parkinsonian syndrome, frequently induces extensive sialorrhoea, occasionally at low dosages (10–25 mg). It can only be diminshed by lowering of dosage.

18.3. Difficulties with visual accommodation

The anticholinergic effect of many psychotropic drugs can give rise to mydriasis and particularly disorders of visual accommodation. The patients complain of difficulties in reading, knitting, and adapting the eyes to small objects. In severe cases there is even a blurring of vision looking at remote objects. This side effect is sometimes disturbing, but mainly for intellectual patients whose reading is impaired. The effect is reversible and disappears quickly after cessation of treatment. See **19**. The blurred vision is created by a relaxation of the ciliary muscles. Some of the antipsychotic drugs induce pupillary constriction, others dilation.

In cases of glaucoma, especially of the narrow-angle type, the anticholinergic effect requires close supervision by an ophthalmologist. Caution is necessary, but we do not consider glaucoma an absolute contraindication, despite the position taken by other authors (5, 51, 131, 178). The problem rises frequently because depression is very common in older age groups where glaucoma is common. Up to now there exist no antidepressant drugs wholly free of anticholinergic effects.

Minor tranquilizers can be administered without difficulties. Although the exacerbation of symptoms of glaucoma may be infrequent, they are always a serious complication and should be kept in mind and checked on.

18.4. Tachycardia and bradycardia

Tachycardia has already been mentioned as a side effect of the anticholinergic and adrenergic actions of psychotropic drugs and can be connected with palpitation. Bradycardia is frequently seen in treatment with reserpine (which is rarely administered today).

18.5. Urinary retention

Micturition difficulty as a side effect of psychotropic drugs is more frequent than reported. Many patients do not complain spontaneously, and if in the milder cases the doctor does not look for this side effect he will not find it. Patients may suffer from incomplete micturition, frequent micturition, or even complete inhibition. The mechanism of action is not clear, because in theory the anticholinergic effect should relax the detrusor muscle and contract the sphincter muscle of the bladder (28).

The vesical dysfunction induced by major tranquilizers may also be due to competitive inhibition of acetylcholine at the neuromuscular junction of the detrusor pelvic nerves. The degree of dysfunction is related to dosage, duration of drug ingestion, and the individual patient's susceptibility (148). If the diagnosis is missed and the disturbance is not treated by an injection of dihydroergotamine, the patient may needlessly be repeatedly catheterized. If the diagnosis is made early enough, catheterization can usually be avoided. Most susceptible to such disturbances are elderly patients, especially men with prostatic hypertrophy. During psychotropic drug treatment one has to look for early symptoms of inhibition of micturition and to counteract these with dihydroergotamine in doses of ten to twenty drops, t.i.d.

18.6. Perspiration

Perspiration is a frequent autonomic side effect seen with antidepressants, antipsychotics, and minor tranquilizers. In some cases one can observe an excessive sweating of the upper half of the body or the face, preponderantly during the night but sometimes also in the form of acute attacks during the day. There seems to be some correlation of sweating and favorable response to imipramine (216).

18.7. Body temperature

Phenothiazines have been used to induce *hypothermia* and it is obvious that many of these drugs can lower body temperature. Hypothermia is not usually of any clinical importance, but *hyperthermia* is. It may be the first symptom or sign of a central intoxication with potentially lethal consequences. It is a known side effect of strong antipsychotic drugs and should be a warning to reduce the dose. If this is not done, hyperpyrexia may be complicated by increased neurological excitability, cloudiness of consciousness, coma, and death. The slight increase of body temperature frequently seen during antipsychotic drug treatment is without clinical relevance.

19. VISUAL

The autonomic effects (see **18.3.**) can induce miosis, mydriasis, and other disturbances of accommodation.

Some medications, notably antiparkinsonian drugs, lead to weakness of the muscles of visual accommodation. This makes it difficult to focus in near vision whereas distance vision is less frequently affected. Patients should be forewarned of this, since they may otherwise feel they have developed some serious brain pathology.

There also exists the risk of exacerbating a preexisting glaucoma (see **18.3**). Of special interest are pigmentary changes of the eyes. Long-term medication, especially phenothiazines in high dosages, can induce pigmentation not only of the skin but of the eyes. Changes have been observed in the anterior part of the lens and less frequently in the endothelium of the cornea. Changes of the cornea occur after those of the lens. One can also observe pigmentation of the conjunctiva and the anterior surface of the iris. Although axial changes of the eyes are very frequent in the normal population— they can be found in 10 percent of people over forty years of age (135)—there is no doubt that they also can be a consequence of phenothiazines. The side effect has been proven by a controlled study (60) and is partly reversible (74). The pigmentations are dose-related to the cumulative doses and therefore to duration of administration of the medication. Furthermore, a genetic disposition and hormonal and race-related factors seem to contribute, as demonstrated by the fact that blacks have a higher incidence (64). It is important to realize that the patient himself will experience no subjective discomfort and hence will not complain. The physician must look for this side effect.

Attempts to treat the condition with D-penicillamin (84) have met with dubious success, although Greiner and coworkers report considerable improvement in abnormal pigmentation due to chlorpromazine with the use of this drug (D-penicillamin), by avoidance of direct sunlight, by a low copper diet, and by injections of melatonin. The changes of lens and cornea are sometimes associated with photosensitivity. Fortunately, follow-up studies over three years have shown that the changes are less dangerous than was initially feared (73). However, there is no doubt that in long-term medication with high dosages of antipsychotics ophthalmological examinations are necessary. The side effects have been observed more frequently in the United States because higher dosages of chlorpromazine and thioridazine have been used.

Another important side effect is *retinopathy* resulting from dislocation of pigments. The effects are dose-related and are mainly observed after long-term administration of daily dosages of 600-800 mg or more of thioridazine. Therefore it is preferable to administer depot preparations because the necessary cumulative dosage is considerably lower.

The lens opacities induced by some drugs are the result of an accumulation of deposits of the drugs themselves or of their metabolites. There is also evidence that the pigment is melanin and that schizophrenic patients are more prone to disturbances of melanogenesis (80,81).

20. GASTROINTESTINAL

20.1. Nausea and vomiting

Most of the tricyclic psychotropic drugs have antiemetic properties; chlorpromazine, for instance, has been used extensively in
earlier years for the treatment of hyperemesis gravidarum. Prochlorperazine is a widely used antiemetic. Despite these pharmacological properties, psychotropic drugs can induce nausea or vomiting.
But one has to remember that the same effects are also observed
with placebos. Nausea and vomiting, if they occur at all, are almost
always found during the first days of treatment. The pathogenetic
mechanism is not precisely known, but, since many drugs are
anticholinergic and induce hypomotility and relaxation of the stomach, it may be connected with a dysfunction of motility. A rare but
important complication of reserpine treatment is perforation of
gastric ulcers. The symptoms may be hidden by the medication, and
the complication may lead to lethal consequences. Therefore, a
previous medical history of gastric or duodenal ulcer is a near
absolute contraindication for reserpine. On the other hand, a direct
central nervous action has also to be considered, because nausea
and vomiting are frequently associated with dizziness.

20.2. Dryness of the mucosa

See **18.1.**, **18.1.1.**, **18.1.2.**, and **18.1.3.**

20.3. Constipation

Constipation is a frequent symptom in the normal population and especially during psychiatric illnesses. It is one of the most frequent symptoms of depression and can also be induced by tension and anxiety. Unfortunately, the anticholinergic action of antidepressant drugs may elevate this symptom to a severe dysfunction. The constipation has frequently been treated by a laxative (for instance, Dulcolax). It is important to ask carefully for details of the constipation because many patients complain in spite of the fact that they have normal function. The constipation is frequently associated with a reduction of gastric secretion and in the most severe cases one can observe a paralytic ileus. Autopsies of psychiatric patients showed a 12 percent dilatation of one or several parts of the intestine compared to a control group with only 2 percent. The dilatation is a consequence of chronic constipation induced by the anticholinergic action.

20.4. Diarrhea

Diarrhea is a rare side effect of psychotropic drugs. It is especially frequent during the initial period of lithium treatment and can be prevented by slow increase of the dosage. Overdosage of psychotropic drugs in elderly patients may lead to incontinence (115).

21. BODY WEIGHT AND HEIGHT

An increase of body weight during pharmacotherapy is frequently observed. Depressed patients often suffer from loss of appetite and weight, and clinical improvement is correlated with an increase of both. Some authors describe a positive correlation between increase of body weight and clinical response (101, 213, 217). An increase of body weight is frequently observed during long-term treatment with antipsychotics. Some drugs seem especially to induce an increase of appetite, for instance, maprotiline. This may also be true for depot preparations. A loss of body weight can be associated with a worsening of the condition. During lithium treatment increase of body weight is a very important side effect. There does not exist a specific treatment of this sometimes uncomfortable phenomenon. It is not only a consequence of reduction of motility or activity of the patient, since it occurs not only in hospitals but appears to be a true slowing of vital functioning. A few drugs have been reported to decrease body weight occasionally, for instance, molindone and fluspirilene. Treatment of hyperactive children by dextroamphetamine or methylphenidate is reported to induce a highly significant suppression of growth in weight and height (187). Tolerance develops to the weight suppressant effect but not to the inhibition of height and growth.

22. HEPATIC

Changes of hepatic functions are shown by a decrease or increase of bilirubin in the blood, by transitional increase of transaminases or alkaline phosphatase, and, rarely, by the occurrence of jaundice. A slight decrease of bilirubin has been described, for instance, during treatment with thioridazine (102) and may frequently be missed. Perhaps there is some inhibition of synthesis of bilirubin.

There is an extensive literature on hepatoxicity of phenothiazines, especially chlorpromazine, but there is no proof for the assumption that the latter is more toxic than other substances. As a rule jaundice, if it is to occur at all, develops within the first three months of the treatment. Prodromal symptoms lasting about two weeks are fever, nausea, gastric pains, and dizziness. Jaundice itself lasts on the average about three weeks in conjunction with anorexia, weakness, tiredness, pruritus, alcholic excrements, dark urine, and occasionally enlargement of the liver. Alkaline phosphate and the bromsulphalein-test are abnormal. Sometimes cholesterol in the blood is increased. SGOT is increased but not as high as during a viral hepatitis. The serum proteins are usually normal, and the blood eosinophile count occasionally is elevated. Histologically there is a picture of biliary stasis with biliary thromboses in the canaliculi. The stasis is most marked in the centrolobular region; the portal region is infiltrated by mononuclear cells, lymphocytes, and, frequently, eosinophilic cells. Occasionally there is some degeneration or necrosis of liver cells. Investigations by electron microscope (208) show abnormalities in the microvilli and along the canaliculi.

There seems to be no correlation between dosage and the risk of jaundice. The frequency of jaundice during drug treatment is difficult to estimate because there is also coincidence of the two purely by chance. If such cases are included, the incidence is about 2 percent.

Much more frequent than jaundice are transitional changes of liver enzymes that last only a few weeks. Symptoms and signs decrease despite continued drug treatment. Such changes have also been found in children, not only during treatment with chlorpromazine or similar compounds but also with minor tranquilizers. The prognosis for liver changes and for jaundice is usually favorable. An interesting double-blind study (103) compared twenty patients on chlorpromazine with twenty-five on placebos. The changes were the same in quantity and quality in both groups. Biopsies showed fatty infiltration, portal fibrosis, and proliferation in the biliary tracts.

23. HEMATOLOGICAL

23.1. Agranulocytosis

There is a wide range of hematological effects of psychotropic drugs ranging from leukopenia to agranulocytosis. The latter is very rare and is most frequently found when psychotropics are combined with other medications such as barbiturates. There is no indication for the assumption that some of the drugs are more prone than others to induce agranulocytosis. The symptoms of agranulocytosis are local infection, fever, pharyngitis, ulceration, dysphagia, dermatitis, enterocolitis, and sometimes jaundice. Fortunately the prognosis is usually good. After cessation of the medication the changes are frequently reversible within two weeks. The prognosis is much better, for instance, than in aplastic anemia induced by chloramphenicol. The treatment is conservative and consists of giving antibiotics. The mortality rate for agranulocytosis is 10 to 20 percent. There is some disagreement as to the usefulness of routine blood tests. We consider this important only initially (for two months) and after that useless. The increase of agranulocytosis correlates with the cumulative dosage of phenothiazines.

23.2. Leukopenia

Leukopenia is much more frequent than agranulocytosis and does not produce clinical symptoms. In one three-month trial in which leukocytes were monitored weekly, six of sixteen subjects showed some leukopenia. On the other hand, Turunen and Salminen (228) compared 273 patients who had been treated by antipsychotic drugs with a control group of 248 patients. The mortality in the first group was 11 percent and in the second 11.6 percent, a result of no statistical significance. Two patients died of agranulocytosis.

About twice as common as agranulocytosis, leukopenia can be observed in children, though older patients are especially prone to develop the condition. It seems to occur more frequently in females than in males, but then psychotropics are more frequently prescribed for females. White patients may possibly develop leukopenia more frequently than blacks (59).

23.3. Eosinophilia

Eosinophilia is very frequent, especially during the first few weeks of treatment with psychotropic drugs. It has no clinical significance. Imipramine treatment, for instance, can provoke a rise in the eosinophile count in 4–7 percent of cases. In a double-blind trial there was an increase of eosinophilia in 18 percent of patients receiving a placebo and in 37 percent of those treated with imipramine (139). Eosinophilia may occur in children as well as adults.

23.4. Anemia and purpura

Fatal aplastic anemia has been observed in a patient on lithium (107). It is uncertain what role the drug played in the condition. There is some evidence for a biochemical defect in the marrow cells of chlorpromazine sensitive patients (164). Vascular purpura is a very rare side effect of psychopharmeceuticals (123).

23.5. E.S.R.

A rise in the erythrocyte sedimentation rate is frequently observed during the first weeks of psychotropic medication. It is sometimes accompanied by a slight transient increase of the white blood count. The changes are not of clinical significance.

23.6. Coagulation

There is some evidence that chlorpromazine and other drugs may inhibit coagulation and increase the anticoagulation properties of the blood. In a second phase there may be hypercoagulation. The first phase seems to be due to hemolysis of the erythrocytes or to inhibition of the thrombocyte phosphodiesterase (157, 185).

23.7. Thromboembolia

During psychotropic drug treatment the risk of thromboembolia is increased. Meier-Ewert and coworkers (146) found 2.9 percent complications in a sample of 1,172 patients compared to a control group with 0.6 percent. The risk is higher in females than in males. Predisposing factors are varicosites, cardiac insuffiency, and fever. In some cases the thromboses can be complicated by a fatal pulmonary embolus. There is no doubt that the risk of thromboses is increased by psychotropic drug treatment. The most important factor is immobilization of the patient, especially if the inexperienced doctor prescribes bed rest. On the other hand, there also may be an increased stasis of the peripheral circulation related to edema of the legs. These edemae are mainly seen after activity, e.g., if the patient has had to stand more than usual during work therapy. They are not a consequence of cardiac insufficiency but of venostasis.

24. DERMATOLOGICAL

Skin reactions as a side effect of psychotropic drugs are not unusual but they are rarely severe. Chlorpromazine and other phenothiazines can create a *photosensitivity* of the skin. Therefore those parts of the body that are exposed to sunlight may show skin reactions. Simple *allergic reactions* in the form of urticaria, erythema, or maculopapular rashes can be observed. A photosensitive patient can be protected by the application of a benzophenone lotion.

A thorough study by Jung et al. (112) showed a cross-sensitivity with respect to different psychopharmaceuticals. They suggest that the photoallergy responsible for such skin reactions may be due to chromatic transformation products which are produced upon exposure to ultraviolet light. Chiefly implicated in this connection are products of dimerization which, since they are insoluble, remain at the site of their formation, i.e., in the skin. The resultant permanent contact between these substances and the skin promotes epidermal sensitization and also accounts for the chronic recurrent character of such photodermatoses. Fortunately, however, these skin reactions usually disappear after psychoactive drug therapy has been withdrawn. Very rarely, one can observe skin lesions reminiscent of lupus erythematosus or exfoliative dermatitis. A causal connection has not been established.

The most important dermatological side effects are *pigmentations* of a grey or metallic color. They are a consequence of long-term medication with phenothiazines or similar compounds in high dosages. The pigmentations are located in sun-exposed parts of the body and are frequently associated with pigmentation of the eyes. Histologically there is an increased pigmentation in the basic layers of the skin with a depot in the dermis. Occasionally the skin produces a glimmer of blue (Tyndall-effect). These patients have been referred to as "purple people." An increased production of melanin in the epidermis has been found without any clinical signs of pigmentation (182). Patients with pigmentation of the skin show an altered metabolism of chlorpromazine in favor of hydroxylation and conjugation; the formation of glucoronides seems to be inhibited because there is less conjugated chlorpromazine in the urine (4, 45). There is no correlation between pigmentation of the skin and neurological (232) or gastroenterological effects (234). Lee and coworkers (130) have raised an interesting hypothesis of a connection between orthostatic hypotension, extrapyramidal symptoms, and ocular and skin pigmentation. They think that a drug which induces decrease of catecholamines thereby produces orthostatic hypotension, an increase of MSH and a decreased synthesis of melatonin. The latter induces an increased activity of melanocytes in the eyes, skin, and brain stem. A massive dosage of phenothiazines exhausts the melanocytes in the epidermis, the pigment descends into the dermis, and the overflow of melanin, together with the overflow of chlorpromazine, forms a complex which constitutes the observed pigmentation.

25. ENDOCRINOLOGICAL

25.1. Galactorrhea and gynecomastia

Galactorrhea and gynecomastia are infrequent side effects of psychotropic drugs. The problem has received special attention from Shader and DiMascio (207). They stress that squeezing the nipple may reveal the presence of galactorrhea in some subjects in whom it might otherwise go unrecognized. Some patients complain of increasing size of the breasts, tension, and occasionally galactorrhea. A mammotropic effect of many substances has been shown in rats (chlorpromazine, thioridazine, trifluoperazine, prochlorperazine, fluphenazine, imipramine, amitriptyline, meprobamate, chlorprothixene, thiothixene, haloperidol, chlordiazepoxide, and many other drugs).

The side effect is more frequent with long-term use of medication in high dosages. In females it is often connected with amenorrhea, occasionally also with decrease of libido (140). The side effect can be corrected by reduction of dosage or change to another preparation. Kolpocytological investigations show in cases of galactorrhea a disturbed balance of estrogens. The mechanism may be due partly to inhibition of the secretion of prolactin in the pituitary or possibly to direct influence on the hypothalamus. Shader and DiMascio think it probable that galactorrhea is caused by suppression of the secretion of a prolactin-inhibitory factor in the hypothalamus (median eminence).

25.2.Amenorrhea

Menstrual irregularities are very common in psychiatric disorders (schizophrenia, depression, mania, neuroses). However, changes during drug treatment have yet to be monitored by predrug evaluations. The mechanism is not clear. There are arguments for a drug effect on the hypothalamus or on the pituitary gland; others suggest also end-organ inhibition as the cause of amenorrhea. Amenorrhea can be associated with galactorrhea. Some studies indicate elevated values of FSH and estrone. Menstrual irregularities or amenorrhea have been reported as side effects of most of the psychotropics. But, as mentioned above, the interpretation has to take into account that the same symptom is also found in the psychiatric disorder itself. The occurrence of this side effect is grounds for recommending a gynecological examination to exclude other causes. There is no specific treatment to suggest and the condition is benign.

25.3. Effects on the hypothalamic-pituitary-adrenal axis

Investigations in this field are very controversial. The results have been summarized by Shader and coworkers (207a). They suggest that chlorpromazine may depress ACTH-secretion by acting on the hypothalamus (inhibition of CRF) and by acting on the pituitary (inhibition of the release of ACTH) or by blocking the susceptibility of the pituitary to CRF.

25.4. Thyroid

Most of the psychotropic drugs do not effect thyroid functions. Generally observed disturbances are primary and the psychiatric disorder is secondary. The literature on drug-induced thyroid dysfunction is controversial and no conclusion can be drawn. One has to assume that a specific effect has not been shown (205). The only drug that has definitely been shown to interfere with thyroid function is lithium.

Most but not all lithium data are consistent with the following mode of action. The initial effects are (a) partial inhibition of thyroid uptake of iodide; (b) partial inhibition of thyroid hormone release from the gland; and (c) a decrease in the peripheral hormone degradation rate in some patients. Subsequently, as the peripheral hormone level drops, negative feedback results in increased TSH production, resulting in an increase in the thyroid clearance of iodide. This increase builds up the intrathyroidal iodine pool until, even though the fractional release rate remains reduced, the intra-thyroidal iodine pool increases to a point where the absolute amount of iodine released per unit of time approximates the predrug level. Thus it appears that, provided a normal gland is present and able to compensate for its changed environment, the patient remains euthy-roid, although with changed iodine kinetics.

25.5. LH and GH

Plasma lutenizing hormone (LH) and estrogens and growth hor-mones (GH) were measured during neuroleptic treatment without the discovery of any significant change (29, 30, 191). Of female patients with inappropriate breast activity and/or amenorrhea under phenothiazines, most had an elevated plasma prolaction (30) that fell to within the normal range upon cessation of the drug treatment and rose again when it was reinstated. Immunoelectrophoretic analyses have shown that the secretion of the male mammary glands is a specific one very similar to normal but differing in some respects (129).

25.6. Diabetes insipidus

Long-term lithium treatment can induce a temporary renal dia-betes insipidus which is vasopressin resistant. Lithium inhibits the adenylcyclase that transforms ATP into cyclic ATP which, in turn, increase ADH (antidiuretic hormone). Therefore about 12 percent of the patients on lithium show a lowered ability to conserve water. In 3 percent there is a lowered ability to conserve sodium (Na). The latter is dangerous because the daily need for sodium is increased, and the lithium clearance may decrease and lithium accumulate in the blood so that the patient becomes intoxicated. The symptoms of this intoxication are similar to adrenal insufficiency but the mineral corticoids are not decreased. Lithium intoxications due to this mechanism are rare; the exact frequency is not known.

25.7. Sexual function

Psychotropic drugs may have as a side effect decreased libido, impotence, and disturbed ejaculation. Shader (201, 202) suggested that hypothalamic sympathetic depression and peripheral alpha-adrenergic blockade could be the underlying mechanisms for ejaculation disorders. Also the motility of sperm may be changed. Changes of spermatogenesis and ejaculation have been reported as side effects of reserpine, trifluoperazine, perphenazine, butyrylperazine, trifluperidol (35), and mesoridazine (204). Difficulties of ejaculation have been observed in males taking thioridazine, chlorprothixene, pargyline, and chlordiazepoxide. Minor tranquilizers in general, as is the case with many antipsychotic drugs, can reduce libido and potency. On the other hand, MAO-inhibitors (phenelzine) seem to stimulate semen volume (Davis et al. [51a]). Long-term medication has not yet been shown, to influence gonadotropin excretion or sperm production to a significant degree. Priapism seems to be a very rare side effect (40).

25.8. Glucose metabolism

Psychiatric patients in general have levels of blood sugar higher than the average for normal populations (206). Up to now there is no agreement upon the question of whether psychotropic drugs can induce a diabetes mellitus or not. Phenothiazines may have a hyperglycemic effect in certain patients; antidepressants may lower the blood sugar. It is not yet clear whether we are dealing with changes of the threshold or whether the medication can provoke the manifestation of a latent or prediabetic condition. The literature on diabetes and chlorpromazine has been reviewed by Korenyi and Lowenstein (122).

26. PREGNANCY AND PUERPERIUM

From a methodological point of view it is extremely difficult to establish *teratogenic effects* of drug treatment, especially if the risk is very low. Since the disaster of thalidomide all researchers in this field have become aware of this danger in the development of new drugs. Despite such continuous awareness there is as yet no evidence to suggest that any psychotropic drug currently on the market increases the usual rate of malformations. The single cases that have been reported do not allow us to draw any conclusions. In the face of the worldwide use of psychotropic drugs, reports on malformations after drug treatment are extremely rare and the incidence is not significant. For instance, the review of Ayd (16) on eight years of perphenazine use concludes that there is no evidence of malformations despite the fact that about twenty-five million patients have been treated by the drug. Reviewing the use of chlorpromazine (17, 18) he comes to the same conclusion. The review of Shader (203) and the report of Van Waes and Van de Velde (233) do not show any elevated risk of teratogenesis. One has to point out again that the antiemetic action of psychotropic drugs (especially chlorpromazine and—demonstrated more recently—haloperidol) is such that they have been widely used for the treatment of hyperemesis gravidarum (233). The conclusion is that there is no scientific evidence for the assumption that any psychotropic drug on the market can induce malformations of newborn children. On the other hand, the research methods used cannot completely exclude the risk. The general medical rule is still valid that we should if possible avoid any drugs during the first trimester of pregnancy. The question is especially important in cases of long-term treatment because here the probability of treating a pregnant woman is much higher.

Schou and coworkers (195, 196, 197) have summarized our knowledge on *lithium and pregnancy*. This review is especially important because there is strong evidence for an inhibition of synthesis of thyroxine by lithium and one could expect an increase risk of hypothyroidism in lithium babies. Some cases have been reported but in the face of known spontaneous occurrence a causal relationship has not been established. Schou and coworkers published investigations of 118 lithium babies. Of these, five were stillborn, seven died within the first week of life, and six of these twelve children were malformed. The total number of malformations was nine (two children with Down's syndrome); in six of nine cases there was malformation of the cardiovascular system. The conclusion is: "The risk of teratogenic effects is lower than one might have expected from some of the studies carried out on rats and mice; they do not answer the question of whether or not lithium is teratogenic in man" (195).

On the other hand, there is agreement on the fact that drugs given to the mother during labor or in the lactation period pass the placenta and enter into the blood of the fetus or enter into the maternal milk. The application of minor tranquilizers during labor can induce a sedation of the newborn (33, 72). The application of psychotropic drugs or barbiturates can induce a depression of respiration over days and in some cases even a persistent sedation of behavior for months (55). Extrapyramidal side effects after treatment of the mother with a major tranquilizer were found in one case of a neonate for as long as six months (97). Newborn infants are reported to show occasional respiratory, circulatory, and neurological symptoms after imipramine treatment of the mother during pregnancy (62, 63). The following drugs have been found in the milk of the mother: chlorpromazine (229), chlordiazepoxide in minimal amounts, diazepam, meprobamate, and lithium. A summary was given by Ayd (20).

27. MINERAL METABOLISM

Lovett-Doust and Huszka (136) assume that the effect of phenothiazines and butyrophenones is to increase plasma potassium and the plasma corticoids. The administration of phenelzine can lead to an increase in plasma sodium and a fall in magnesium.

28. PHOSPHOLIPIDS

A new psychotropic side effect that has to be investigated in the future is a change of phospholipid metabolism (137).

29. SUDDEN DEATH DURING DRUG TREATMENT

It is very well known that acute schizophrenic psychoses, especially catatonia, can be lethal. An analysis of seventeen cases by Dynes (57) showed that only five of these patients had been treated by phenothiazines. A more recent review by Peele and Loetzen (162) raised doubts as to the validity of phenothiazine death as an entity. Considering the world wide consumption of psychotropic drugs the reports on lethal complications are extremely rare and may often be coincidental. In a small proportion of the cases there may be a partial causality connected with treatment, for instance, in cases of cardiovascular side effects (25, 153). A thorough investigation by Moore and Book (153) of seventy-five deaths after pheonthiazine treatment showed that autopsies did not provide significant findings to explain the death. The authors offer as possible mechanisms the possiblity of cardiovascular reactions or asphyxia or an interference with autonomic regulation or autoimmune reactions or a particular susceptibility to phenothiazines. Extremely few of the cases are definitely due to psychotropic drug treatment such as lethal agranulocytosis or hepatitis (228) or anaphylactic shock after chlorpromazine (186) or embolisms after thromboses (132).

Summarizing the literature, one has to conclude that there is no concrete evidence on which to assume that psychotropic drugs give rise to an increased mortality. On the contrary there is a great deal of evidence for the assumption that the administration of drug treatment lowers the otherwise lethal course of some schizophrenic psychoses, and the risk of suicide is substantially diminished. Deaths from manic exhaustion have virtually disappeared.

A study of Matsuki and coworkers (144) shows that schizophrenic patients on long-term phenothiazine treatment may have a higher morbidity and mortality in cases of emergency abdominal surgery if the anesthesiologists and surgeons are not aware of the risk. A comparative study of patients with cardiac disease on amitriptyline treatment as compared to a control group showed no difference in terms of mortality with or without the amitriptyline. On the other hand, in the amitriptyline group there was an increased risk of sudden death in patients seventy years and older (151).

30. NEUROLOGICAL

Neurological side effects of psychotropic drugs, excluding the autonomic nervous system, are listed below.

30.1. Tremor

Antipsychotic and antidepressent drugs may induce a slight or coarse tremor without any extrapyramidal side effects. The same is true for long-term lithium treatment. Tremor can be very disturbing for the patient and has to be treated by antiparkinsonian medication. Lithium tremor is difficult to control. Claims have been made that the condition may be influenced by the application of beta-blocking agents such as propanolol (80 mg per day). Others have advocated clozapine, tryptophane, etc.

30.2. Parkinsonian syndrome

The parkinsonian syndrome is characterized by akinesia and rigidity. The full clinical picture is very well known. During drug treatment one can observe micrographia as an early symptom; its occurrence has been used to determine the threshold of effective doses (Haase [85]). A number of authors thought that extrapyramidal effects of antipsychotic drugs were a necessary condition to induce antipsychotic activity. Newer investigations have shown that there is no correlation between clinical effect and parkinsonian reactions. New drugs with remarkable antipsychotic activity may have no, or practically no, extrapyramidal activity (clozapine, lenperone). There is no evidence for the assumption that antiparkinsonian medication will decrease the clinical effectiveness of antipsychotic drugs. On the other hand, it is obvious that for the patient the parkinsonian syndrome places a severe restriction not only on motility but also on psychological behavior, contact with others, and mental activity (bradyphrenia). The patient becomes slow, speaks in a monotone, at times can't speak loudly enough, and so on. The parkinsonian syndrome should therefore be avoided as far as possible by reduction of dosages or additional antiparkinsonian medication.

Extrapyramidal side effects are observed more frequently in antipsychotic drugs (tricyclic substances) with piperazinylalcyl side chains and also in butyrophenones. They are less frequent in phenothiazines with aliphatic side chains. On the other hand, there is also some negative correlation with the sedative effect of antipsychotic drugs. The less sedative a drug is, the more frequent in general are extrapyramidal effects. The extrapyramidal activity in humans shows a high correlation to the catatonic effect in animals. Some patients may show a persistent parkinsonian syndrome after cessation of drug treatment. Ayd (15) has shown that the age distribution of these patients is the same as for those with spontaneous parkinsonism. One has therefore to assume that in these patients the drug treatment coincides with the manifestation of paralysis agitans or may precipitate the onset of the disorder. Cessation of drug treatment may sometimes lead to a temporary increase in extrapyramidal symptomatology. This is due to a slower elimination of antipsychotic than of antiparkinsonian drugs. Antiparkinsonian drugs should be continued for a week after discontinuance of the major tranquilizers. Tricyclic antidepressants are anticholinergic agents and act as antiparkinsonian drugs. Alone, they do not usually induce extrapyramidal side effects, though parkinsonism has been observed with high doses of amitriptyline. Imipramine, for instance, has been widely used for the treatment of Parkinson's disease. The incidence of extrapyramidal side effects appears lower in combinations of perphenazine with amitriptyline than with perphenazine alone.

30.3. Acute dystonia

During the first few days of antipsychotic treatment, dystonic reactions are most dramatic and important. They should not be mistaken for hysterical attacks. In decreasing frequency, from head to feet, acute muscle spasms can be observed: for instance, oculogyric crises (the patient having a fixed upward gaze), spasms of the tongue (retracted or extended), spasms of the lips or face (grimaces), torticollis, neck twisting, spasms of the arms or legs. The crises are frequently unilateral. Opisthotonus is unfortunately sometimes misdiagnosed as hysteria. These side effects are more frequent on nonsedative antipsychotic drugs and butyrophenones than on phenothiazines with aliphatic side chains.

The treatment by intravenous injection of an antiparkinsonian drug (5 mg Akineton i.v.) is very successful. The attack disappears within seconds. The side effect is no reason for the interruption of treatment but one has to add an oral antiparkinsonian drug daily. Younger patients are more susceptible than older ones, and males are more prone than females. The risk of dystonic reactions during medication with phenothiazines of the piperazine class is so high that it is generally recommended in treating ambulatory patients to start such a drug together with an antiparkinsonian medication for at least the first two weeks.

30.4. Akathisia

Akathisia is a condition in which the patient is not able to sit still. He suffers from restless legs and is forced to stand up and move around. Sitting on a chair or standing, he has to shift his legs continuously. The side effect is very prominent and should not be misdiagnosed as psychotic agitation. The patient often describes his condition as "wanting to get outside of his skin." The treatment is very difficult because antiparkinsonian drugs do not always influence akathisia. In such cases akathisia is an indication for the interruption of treatment and a switch to a different preparation. The condition develops during the first few months of a drug treatment and is mainly seen in middle-aged patients, especially females.

30.5. Persistent dyskinesia (tardive dyskinesia)

Persistent dyskinesia is one of the most important and most severe side effects of antipsychotics. The symptomatology varies greatly from one case to another. The condition develops after months or years of treatment and can persist for years and even after cessation of treatment. Initial appearance may occur either during treatment or after treatment has been discontinued since the drug itself may mask the existence of the side effect. The frequency is variable; some investigations estimate the frequency at more than 30 percent, depending upon how one defines the limits of the disorder.

The most common symptoms are clonic involuntary contractions of single muscles or muscle groups preponderantly around the mouth, movements of the tongue ("fly catching"), licking, lip smacking, blinking, chewing movements, and involuntary movements of fingers, hands, or shoulders. In severe cases there may be hemiballismus or gross movements of the upper part of the body (forwards and backwards). The most dangerous symptom is spasm of the glottis.

The treatment of this severe side effect is very difficult. It is necessary to stop the drug treatment. In some cases one can switch to a major tranquilizer which does not produce such a reaction, for instance, clozapine. Most of the drugs with piperazinyl side chains are able to reduce the movements. Antiparkinsonian drugs are not very effective. Lecithin has been claimed to be useful.

There is a correlation between the risk of persistent dyskinesia and cumulative dosage of neuroleptic drugs. Therefore, in long-term treatment one should reduce the dosage as much as possible. Females are more prone than males, older patients more so than younger, and cases with brain damage especially so. EEG examinations show paroxysmal activities and signs of organic brain damage (161). Studies of control groups have shown that spontaneous persistent dyskinesia is very frequent in older patients and not always a consequence of antispychotic treatment. There is a lack of pathological anatomical investigations in this field. The biochemical mechanism is not known exactly. One proposal is that the stereotyped behavior seen in animals and in human beings, including tardive dyskinesia in man, may be due to an abnormal sensitivity of the striatal dopaminergic receptors to dopamine (116). A blind study showed that L-dopa together with a decarboxylase inhibitor precipitated or aggravated the dyskinesia while AMPT (alpha-methyl-paratyrosine) reduced the symptomatology significantly. The authors concluded that dopaminegic hypersensitivity, cholinergic hypofunction, and reduced biological buffer capacity are important elements in the pathophysiology of tardive dyskinesia. The action of physostigmine was not conclusive. In a study using a placebo control, methylphenidate has been tried resulting in an aggravation of the symptoms (70). Reduction can be achieved, it has been claimed, with dopamine-depleting agents (reserpine, tetrabenazine) (114), by blockade with apomorphine (79) and with piperazinyl phenothiazines (thiopropazate) (50).

Tardive dyskinesia has also been observed in children in relation to impaired learning (145, 166). The mechanism may be similar to that of L-dopa dyskinesia. This may result from excessive inhibition of caudate neurones by dopamine; the mechanism responsible for inactivating excessive extraneuronal dopamine (mainly re-uptake) and intraneuronal dopamine (monoamine-oxidase) are impaired in patients with Parkinson's disease. Treatment of Parkinson's disease with L-dopa may induce excessive levels of dopamine at receptor sites, a condition resulting in dyskinesias. Long-term use of neuroleptics causes accelerated production of dopamine, which may continue even after the offending drug is stopped. When brain damage (including loss of dopaminergic fibers to the caudate nucleus) coexists, there is disturbance of dopamine in activation similar to that of Parkinson's disease; the result is increased extracellular dopamine levels and dyskinesia (121).

30.6. Epileptic seizures

Most antipsychotic and antidepressant drugs lower the epileptic threshold and in some cases where there is a special predisposition to epilepsy may provoke epileptic seizures. The side effect is rare but it has been observed during treatment with chlorpromazine, fluphenazine, fluphenazine decanoate, haloperidol, penfluridol, spirioperidol, sulpirid, clozapine, clomacranphosphate, thiothixene, and imipramine. In these cases the drug treatment has to be stopped or replaced by another compound. For the treatment of epileptic psychoses, major tranquilizers may be indicated in spite of these unfavorable actions, and the small epileptogenic effect can be counteracted easily by the administration of an antiepileptic drug. In such cases the physician should prescribe a combination of both. Epileptic seizures have also been observed in children (69).

31. PSYCHOLOGICAL

Undesirable psychotropic effects are listed below.

31.1. Oversedation

Most of the psychotropic drugs are sedative. Even psychostimulant drugs like amphetamines or psychic energizers such as the MAO-inhibitors may occasionally have a paradoxical sedative action. Tricyclic antidepressants (for instance, imipramine) have a sedative action in at least 10 percent of patients and, given in the evening, can improve sleep remarkably. Other patients, however, may feel stimulated and sleepless if the drug is given in the evening.

Oversedation is a serious side effect in long-term treatment. The patient may become apathetic; complain of tiredness, loss of energy, and loss of interest; and may even appear to be depressed. Such symptoms during long-term treatment are frequent and, though sometimes the expression of a beginning parkinsonian syndrome, are more frequently due to oversedation. They can be improved by reduction of dosage.

31.2. Overactivation

Even so-called sedative psychotropic drugs may on occasion activate a patient and worsen the symptomatology. An agitated depressive patient may become more anxious and excited. The doctor, thinking the dosage insufficient, increases it. The vicious circle goes on in this way. The same is true for psychotic states treated by antipsychotic drugs.

31.3. Undesirable mood changes

Mood changes during drug treatment are depression, mania or dysphoria. *Depression* has frequently been described as a side effect of major tranquilizers. Heinrich described a syndrome of exhaustion that appears after remission of a psychotic episode. This may result from the neuroleptic pharmacotherapy or from psychological reactions of the person to the experience, or it may simply be a residual state of schizophrenia (92, 93). Helmchen and Hippius (94) describe an early depression during the second month of neuroleptic treatment and a so-called late depression after three to four months of treatment. Such episodes are characterized by flat dysphoric syndromes with typical endogenous depressive symptoms, daily fluctuation of the symptomatology, hypochondriacal delusions, and depressed mood. This syndrome does not respond to neuroleptic treatment, and many authors think that the drugs themselves may induce such a side effect. Cessation of the medication is usually followed by an immediate improvement.

Depressive syndromes during drug treatment are described for chlorpromazine, trifluoperazine, thioproperazine, butaperazine, fluphenazine, clopenthixol, molindone, fluphenazine decanoate, fluphenazine enanthate, fluspirilene, and pipothiazine palmitate. Depression has also been described in children (200). Recommendations for the management of this condition are controversial. It is not well established that tricyclic antidepressants are useful. If possible, the neuroleptic drug should be stopped. Some authors think that MAO-inhibitors may have a specific antagonistic action (211).

Up to now there is not enough scientific evidence to assume that a causal connection between antipsychotic drug treatment and depression has been established. This is particularly true since it is well known that depressive symptomatology may follow spontaneous remission of an untreated schizophrenic or schizoaffective episode.

Manic syndromes have frequently been observed during antidepressant treatment with tricyclic antidepressants or with MAO-inhibitors. The switch from depression to mania has been thought to be a predictor of the drug's efficacy. But there are no controlled experiments to show that such a switch is more common during drug treatment than during placebos. Patients with bipolar affective disorders are more prone to develop such a mood swing during a depression treated with drugs.

31.4. Exacerbation or provocation of psychotic symptomatology

Activating drugs (amphetamines, MAO-inhibitors, and tricyclic antidepressants) can provoke schizophrenic symptoms if given to the wrong patient. A quiet schizophrenic patient without apparent delusions can become not only agitated or excited but also develop paranoid delusions and hallucinations. This action has occasionally been used as a diagnostic test to exclude schizophrenia.

31.5. Confusion and delirious states

Organic confusional states are rare complications of psychotropic drug treatment. They are most frequently produced by antiparkinsonian drugs. The patient is disorientated in space and time, shows impairment of memory, impairment of other intellectual functions, impairment of judgment, and may show changes of mood (depression, mania) or even delusional symptoms and hallucinations. Some patients describe the reaction as being like an LSD "trip."

Psychometric investigations (27) have demonstrated that long-term treatment with lithium can occasionally induce loss of concentration, loss of recent memory, and loss of initiative and reactivity. Delirious states occurring during psychotropic drug treatment show the same symptomatology as delirium tremens due to alcoholism. The patient shows a motor hyperactivity with coarse tremor of the extremities, illusions (usually visual), and hallucinations. The patient is overactive and tends to concentrate on his illusions. The condition may last several days to a week. Delirious states can induce a marked improvement after their cessation. Delirious states are more common than confusional states during drug treatment. The delirious states are due mainly to the anticholinergic action (for instance, of tricyclic antidepressants or of some antipsychotic drugs, e.g., thioridazine, methotrimeprazine, chlorpromazine, clozapine). They have to be treated by withdrawal of the drug and application of DHE together with chlormethiazole or some equivalent treatment.

Part V. Long-Term Management and Prophylaxis

32. NATURAL COURSE OF SCHIZOPHRENIA AND AFFECTIVE DISORDERS

The natural history of schizophrenia and affective disorders is not adequately known, despite the fact that the majority of such cases require long-term care. No model as yet exists which permits accurate prediction of the course of these disorders, although promising attempts toward a mathematical model have been made in the last few years (Angst et al. [8, 9]). Today we can only observe the course of these disorders under treatment, in ignorance of their natural history and therefore of how much the course is modified by treatment. There is no doubt, for instance, that the course of schizophrenia has changed quite a bit during the last few decades. The proportion of chronic severe residual states or of progressive courses of schizophrenia has diminished remarkably (M. Bleuler [37]). By contrast, the onset of schizophrenia has not changed very much, with two-thirds of first episodes starting with acute manifestations and one-third in a chronic way. The change in the further course has been toward the more phasic and less chronic; the prognosis has therefore become more favorable. The reason for this change is certainly the change in treatment methods.

Psychopharmacotherapy has made a great contribution; based on present knowledge, we have to assume that about one-third of schizophrenic psychoses improve spontaneously to the point that they do not require further drug treatment; two-thirds, however, follow a prolonged course, with many of these patients requiring long-term treatment.

The *affective disorders* have also been shown (Angst et al. [6, 9]) to be highly recurrent. The so-called single episode patients are extremely rare, as can be seen by following these patients over decades. Of course, not every recurrent affective disorder requires prolonged medication. The disorder must be severe enough to justify long-term treatment. Today the criteria for treatment are social. The probability of serious recurrence must be so high that the disadvantage of long-term treatment is less than the disadvantage of recurrence. Usually patients are given long-term treatment if their affective disorder recurs at least once a year. Studies of the course of previously hospitalized patients have shown that this is usually the case after the first few episodes. It is difficult to estimate the proportion of patients who really need such long-term medication, but it is certainly far higher than was once believed. One can estimate that 0.5 percent of the population are suffering from schizophrenia with unfavorable prognosis and that at least 1.5 percent have affective disorders which will recur frequently. These figures suggest the importance of long-term treatment today.

The need for beds for schizophrenic patients has decreased in all Western countries. Strömgren (222) has shown that forty years ago three-fourths of the schizophrenic patients identified in an epidemiological investigation were hospitalized in psychiatric institutions or in nursing homes and only one-fourth were not institutionalized. Today only about a fourth of all schizophrenics are found in institutions. This impressive finding characterizes very well the change in the prognosis of schizophrenia. Gross and coworkers (83) found in a new investigation (1973) that about 25 percent of all schizophrenic psychoses remit completely, 35 percent show characteristic residual states, and 40 percent develop more or less uncharacteristically. The prognosis is better for female than for male patients.

33. LONG-TERM TREATMENT WITH SHORT-ACTING ANTIPSYCHOTIC DRUGS

The introduction of antipsychotics has revolutionized inpatient treatment in psychiatric hospitals. Pharmacotherapeutic effects have made possible a new psychosocial development in psychiatry: discharge from the hospital of many patients to ambulatory treatment or treatment in day or night hospitals; free movement within the hospitals; optimistic attitude of staff toward patients; improvement of the whole milieu in psychiatric institutions; improved possibilities for occupational and work therapy; more effective individual and group psychotherapy; and facilitation of rehabilitation.

The ambulatory treatment of discharged schizophrenic patients with drugs can successfully prevent relapses and rehospitalizations. Pharmacotherapy combined with sociotherapy shows an additive effect (100, 193). There is of course an increased readmission rate of these patients, but the total duration of hospitalization is markedly reduced (128). It is important to know that only good medical aftercare and systematic social-psychiatric rehabilitation can provide the patient maximum benefit.

Thorough investigations have shown that the full therapeutic effect of long-term medication takes three to six months to develop (141) and also after cessation of treatment it may take three to six months for deterioration of the patient's condition to occur (56). Placebo-controlled studies of treatment discontinuance show clearly that long-term medication is very effective (154, 172).

The effect of long-term medication depends, of course, on the regularity of the administration of the psychotropic drug (235). The therapeutic effect depends also on the cooperation of relatives (1, 111, 124, 180, 237) and on social psychiatric rehabilitation (3, 71, 98, 99, 124, 134, 180, 237). The acceptance of medication by the patient depends on the doctor-patient relationship; simply giving the drug may be insufficient. The treatment by a personal doctor gives better results than ambulatory treatment at an outpatient institution (177).

There is no doubt that the daily application of an antipsychotic is in general highly effective in preventing relapses, thereby augmenting rehabilitation, although not every patient profits from this regimen (239). In addition, some patients feel strongly sedated or incapacitated by the medication and are not willing to continue in treatment. Relapses may follow, although this is also true, though less frequently, for patients on long-term medication. Reduction of dosage can also be dangerous and provoke relapses (77). The prognosis depends in part on the spontaneous long-term course of the disorder.

A very difficult question, not yet investigated, is that of the duration of long-term medication in schizophrenia. There is some evidence for the assumption that the most effective period is the first year and that after that the course does not differ very much from placebo-treated control groups (56, 66, 67). In a five-year study it was found that after thirty months the readmission rates no longer differed for drug-treated and the placebo-treated groups (68). At the moment there are no strict rules that can determine how long a patient should be kept on medication. The decision must be made individually, taking into account the actual symptomatology, the reaction of the patient to a lower dosage, and the whole development of the disorder. As long as there are effective symptoms (mood changes) or productive schizophrenic symptoms (delusions, hallucinations) long-term medication is indicated. The same is true in the presence of behavior disturbances.

The choice of antipsychotic drugs. Any antipsychotic drug can be given as a long-term medication, but in many cases the nonsedative compounds are preferable because they are better accepted by the patient. On the other hand, these drugs may provoke more serious extrapyramidal side effects and necessitate long-term medication with antiparkinsonian agents. When prescribing a long-term medication, one should give the lowest possible effective dosage because high dosages may increase the risk of side effects (persistent dyskinesia, persistent parkinsonian syndrome, pigmentation of the eyes and skin, and increase of body weight).

One should also continue to be aware that long-term medication may provoke apathy or even depressive syndromes as side effects. Pharmacotherapy and sociotherapy have an additive effect and in some cases yield results clearly superior to those obtained with placebo-treated groups of schizophrenics (100, 193). An important study by Orlov and coworkers (158) has shown that antiparkinsonian drugs are frequently prescribed unnecessarily during long-term treatment with antipsychotics; often antiparkinsonian medication can be discontinued after a few weeks. Reduction of the antiparkinsonian drug should be attempted. It is also important to note that these same antiparkinsonian drugs can at times produce a toxic (LSD-like) psychosis (often with visual hallucinations) which is then confused with the original condition.

34. LONG-TERM TREATMENT WITH LONG-ACTING ANTIPSYCHOTIC DRUGS

The daily administration of a drug over a period of years presents a great psychological problem. It is very well known that even medications prescribed for a few weeks or months are frequently not taken by the patient. Twenty-five to thirty percent of the medication prescribed in private practice is never taken. The same problem, of course, arises with long-term medication. The fact that once, twice, or even three times a day the patient has to take an antipsychotic drug is a psychological trauma, reminding him day by day that he is a patient. The patient may be very ambivalent in respect to acknowledging the existence of a disorder and the need for treatment, a situation which may induce conflicts with relatives who control the medication, thereby provoking daily arguments which may be disastrous.

There is no doubt that long-acting antipsychotics have great advantages over drugs administered daily. The injection at intervals of one to five weeks does not preoccupy the patient to the same extent as with short-acting drugs. There is not only improvement in the relationship between medical staff and patient, or between relatives and patients, but also a great gain because the daily discussions about drugs are replaced by discussions about the more important problems that the patients have. Relationships may improve dramatically.

A second advantage is that the drug can be administered safely in the prescribed dosage. The risk of relapses is diminished by the intramuscular application of these drugs. Temkov (226) found only a

5 percent relapse rate in the intramuscularly treated group, as compared to 35 percent in the orally-treated group of patients. Imlah and Murphy (108) report a 5 percent relapse rate during fluphenazine decanoate treatment.

There is no doubt that the intramuscular administration of a long-acting antipsychotic agent can improve the prognosis of schizophrenia remarkably. We have reason to hope that we are only at the beginning of this new development and that in the future the prognosis will become even better than in recent decades. Long-term preparations also have *disadvantages*. The therapeutic effect and the side effects may be more evident during the first days or weeks after the injection than just before the next one. In particular, extrapyramidal side effects may be exaggerated immediately after the injection and then gradually improve.

Since we do not have a long-term antiparkinson medication, the patient may be forced to take antiparkinson drugs every day to counteract the side effects of the long-acting medication, thereby losing some of its advantages. The change in degree of side effects may necessitate a continuous change of antiparkinson medication (increase or decrease). This is best done by allowing the patient self-regulation. He should be taught to administer antiparkinson drugs himself. This gives him a feeling of independence and responsibility for his own treatment. It has often been recommended that before starting long-term depot medication an oral form should be administered to test sensitivity to the drug. This may be useful, but the same result can also be obtained by using low dosages of the injectable depot preparation. The dosage of the depot preparation has to be determined individually. The same is true for the interval between injections. The following depot preparations are presently used or are in development:

> Fluphenazine decanoate
> Fluphenazine enanthate
> Fluphenthixol decanoate
> Fluspirilene
> Perphenazine enanthate
> Clopenthixol decanoate
> Pipothiazine palmitate

An interesting development is the introduction of penfluridol (133, 168, 225, 241), an oral long-acting antipsychotic with an effect lasting five to seven days. The once-a-week administration of one or two tablets (20–40 mg) is a promising possibility for long-term treatment and is in many cases preferable to injection.

35. LONG-TERM TREATMENT WITH LITHIUM

Action.   Lithium was introduced in psychiatry by Cade (43) in Australia (1949) for the treatment of mania. It can be given as a long-term treatment for the chronic hypomanic syndrome but much more important is its long-term use as prophylaxis against affective syndromes including depressive ones. It is to the great credit of Hartigan (91) and Baastrup (23) that independently as clinicians they detected the prophylactic effect of lithium. The introduction of lithium as a prophylactic agent is a milestone in modern psychiatry, having dramatically changed the prognosis of affective disorders.

It was the merit of Schou to have confirmed these clinical observations by thorough scientific investigations, first in open and later in double-blind studies. After a lead article in the *Lancet* bearing the title "Lithium, a New Therapeutic Myth" (34), in which the criticism of the pioneering work in lithium was criticized in a rather sophisticated way, further investigations demonstrated that although the methodological arguments were sophisticated they did not arrive at the truth. Today at least eight double-blind studies have been conducted, and all agree that lithium is clearly superior to placebo and can improve the course of affective syndromes. It may in some cases even prevent future episodes. An interruption of a long-term treatment with lithium is followed by a high proportion of relapses (Baastrup et al. [22]). This is true even in patients treated by lithium for many years. It can thus be safely said that the preventive effect does not outlast the period of treatment. The morbidity before, during, and after treatment with lithium has been illustrated in double-blind study by Baastrup and coworkers (22).

Indication. Long-term lithium treatment is indicated in recurrent affective syndromes of depressed, manic, and mixed type, as well as in the schizoaffective syndromes.

The need for treatment depends on the frequency and duration of episodes and the degree of remission in the intervals. Recent studies (Coppen and coworkers [47]) have shown that the so-called free interval of affective syndromes is frequently characterized by hypomanic or subdepressive conditions. One could establish as a general rule that lithium treatment is not indicated if the patient has free intervals of more than one year's duration, if at the same time the episodes do not last longer than a few months and are not so severe as to endanger the patient's life or career. In other words, the treatment is generally indicated if the morbidity persists more than 20–30 percent of the time. A method of estimating the prognosis by taking into account the previous history has been worked out by Angst and coworkers. They show that there is a strong tendency for further relapses and for even shorter intervals between episodes.

The indication for lithium treatment requires a precise diagnosis. Lithium has been shown to have a preventive effect not only in manic-depressive syndromes but also in recurrent depressive ones and, with less efficacy, in schizoaffective disorders. It has not yet been shown to be effective in the recurrent neurotic depressive syndrome. The physician used to prescribing drugs for the treatment of so-called depressive states without a more precise diagnosis will therefore be disappointed.

Administration. Lithium is given as a salt (carbonate, sulfate, citrate, iodide) which is absorbed quickly from the gastrointestinal tract. The serum lithium peak is reached within one to four hours. Gastrointestinal absorption seems to be complete within six to eight hours. For prophylactic purposes one has to reach a serum lithium level of 0.5–1.3 m-equiv./l in healthy adults and slightly less in elderly patients. Lithium is excreted mainly through the kidneys. A normal lithium clearance is therefore necessary to avoid accumulation and intoxication. Before starting lithium treatment, the determination of creatinine or urea in the serum is desirable. The serum level of lithium is usually monitored. Opinion differs as to how frequently this should be done. Some feel it should be determined weekly or twice weekly to adjust dosage during the first two months, with monthly controls for the first year of maintenance as well as one week after every dosage change.

The same is true following significant changes of salt intake. Others believe that serum lithium levels need be taken only if there are clinical indications. A salt-free diet is contraindicated and low salt diets used cautiously during lithium treatment because they may increase renal excretion. Serum lithium levels should be determined on appearance of signs of early toxicity or of relapse, either manic or depressive. Levels may also be changed by the administration of diuretics and should be monitored every week or two if high doses of diuretics are used. When starting lithium treatment we sometimes recommend that dosage be built up gradually within one week because this decreases the frequency of initial side effects.

Clinical effects. Lithium treatment can modify the spontaneous course of affective disorders. It can abbreviate the duration and the amplitude of depressive and manic episodes. It can prolong the duration of intervals (12) and sometimes even prevent future relapses completely. In a minority of cases (10–15 percent) there may be no effect. Patients who have had long-lasting hypomanic intervals may complain of loss of drive, energy, and creativity because they are reduced to normality. In some of these cases the lithium effect may result in a loss for the patient. These are exceptions. In most cases creativity is increased.

Duration of treatment. Our present knowledge suggests that lithium maintenance treatment has to be continued for at least ten years. It is strongly recommended that the patient be given detailed instructions before starting such long-term treatment. The patient must be informed about the future prognosis of the disorder and about the delayed effect of the maintenance therapy: that the prophylactic effect may not become effective for many months and that for a year or two, despite lithium treatment, mild episodes may occur. In general it is preferable, once treatment has been started, to maintain lithium without any discussion during the first year and only after that to decide whether it should be continued. This reinforces the motivation of the patient.

Tolerance.   Lithium in high concentration is a toxic agent and accumulation in the blood must be avoided. Prodromal symptoms of intoxication are diarrhea, vomiting, coarse tremor, fatigue, drowsiness, unsteady gait, and dysarthria. Immediate determination of serum lithium is necessary. The full picture of lithium intoxication is similar to apoplexy (cerebral insult). Clouded consciousness, coma, tremor, myoclonia, muscular hypertonia, increased tendon reflexes, epileptic attacks, changes of EKG, fall of blood pressure, disturbance of water and electrolyte balance, and even shock can occur. Complications can be lethal. Prodromal symptoms of intoxication may occur as a result of altered lithium clearance should nephritis or other intercurrent disorders occur, or as the result of significant reduction of sodium intake or change of treatment with diuretics.

Initial side effects (benign).   Nausea, mild diarrhea, transient tremor of the hands, polydipsia, polyuria.

Late side effects.   Persistent tremor, increased polyuria, polydipsia, increase of body weight, struma, myxedema, edema, and aggravation of acne.

Prevention and treatment of side effects is very important in such long-term treatment. Careful control of the administration of tablets, measurement of serum lithium levels, and monitoring of side effects are all useful and necessary. It is recommended that serum lithium levels be maintained between .6 and 1.0 m equiv./1 if there are side effects. In some cases of persistent side effects it may be necessary to decrease the dosage even more. Tremor of the hands according to reports can be successfully treated by propanolol (40–80 mg daily) or by other beta-receptor blockers. There is no specific treatment for increased body weight, polyuria, and polydipsia. Struma or myxedema are not dangerous and can easily be treated with levothyroxine-natrium (0.1–0.2 mg daily).

Rare side effects of lithium.   Exacerbation of acne vulgaris, allergic skin reactions, exacerbation of psoriasis, leukocytosis, decrease of muscle tonus, unspecific change of EEG, lowering of T-waves in the EKG, decrease of libido or potency. Some patients may complain of loss of concentration and memory. As a rule, this is due to a hidden depression but may also be a consequence of lithium treatment.

Treatment of lithium intoxication. A coma induced by lithium has to be treated similarly to an intoxication by barbiturates. During the first six hours an infusion of saline (1–2 liters) is recommended. In cases of serum levels of more than 4 m equiv./l hemodialysis or peritoneal dialysis is indicated. For further details see Schou (194).

Combination with other drugs. During lithium maintenance treatment hypomanic, manic or depressive episodes may occur. In these cases a combination with tricyclic or tetracyclic antidepressants is necessary. In some cases this may produce increased tremor of the hands necessitating adjustment of the lithium dosage.

36. LONG-TERM TREATMENT WITH ANTIDEPRESSANTS

Experienced clinicians since 1959 (149) have claimed for imipramine a prophylactic action against recurrent depressive disorders. Angst in 1970 (10) summarized the literature of seventeen papers claiming prophylactic action. But the hypothesis of a long-term treatment with a tricyclic antidepressant has never been based on controlled trials until the last few years. A double-blind study by Grof and Vinar (82) in thirty-one patients treated with imipramine in daily doses of 75–100 mg, with placebo, or with neither showed in a sequential analysis no difference among the three groups. Recently, double-blind studies by Kay and coworkers (113) and Mindham and coworkers (150) showed that continuation therapy with tricyclic antidepressants after a good recovery from a depressive episode could benefit as measured by reduced relapse rate. Prien and coworkers (169, 173, 174) showed that a long-term treatment during two years with imipramine gave the same favorable results as lithium treatment in unipolar recurrent depression and was clearly better than placebo treatment. On the other hand, in bipolar manic depressive psychoses imipramine did not affect the manic episodes. An ongoing double-blind trial carried out by Coppen and coworkers (46) shows that long-term treatment with maprotyline, a tetracyclic antidepressant, does not improve the course of bipolar manic depressive syndromes but may have a favorable influence on the course of recurrent depression.

At present a prophylactic effect of long-term treatment with tricyclic or tetracyclic antidepressant compounds is not yet definitively proven but may be of possible use in recurrent depressions. The effect may be comparable to prophylactic treatment with lithium. In bipolar manic depressive syndromes lithium seems preferable.

A long-term treatment with a tricyclic antidepressant may have some advantages over a lithium prophylaxis in regard to toxicity and side-effects. However, we do not as yet know enough to arrive at definitive conclusions.

In some cases a long-term treatment with an antidepressant as a prophylactic agent may be tried in the usual therapeutic dosages (for instance, 150 mg imipramine or amitriptyline or maprotyline). Of course, in these cases the patient also has to be informed about the previous and the expected future course of the disorder and has to be motivated carefully for long-term treatment before beginning.

At times small amounts of antidepressants need to be combined with lithium to keep the patient symptom-free. Hertz and Sulman (96) have also tried to prevent depression with L-tryptophan, but up to now there is not enough evidence to recommend this treatment.

37. LONG-TERM TREATMENT WITH STIMULANTS, MINOR TRANQUILIZERS AND HYPNOTICS

As a general principle it is usually stated that long-term treatment with any member of these three classes of drugs should be avoided. This, however, is not necessarily the case. The reasons why continuing use is cautioned against are: (a) in some patients the drugs have a cumulative effect which produces some impairment of function, and/or (b) tolerance sometimes develops and, in order to obtain a response, the patient or the physician escalates the dose above acceptable limits, and/or (c) the patient may develop a dependence and find it necessary to continue the drug after it is no longer indicated.

If there is no evidence of impairment and no development of tolerance, together with continuing indication for its use, there exists justification for long-term use of either a stimulant, a minor tranquilizer or a hypnotic. Many patients still respond after years of daily use. The drug action appears to be a real one since many times they do not obtain any effect from a substituted placebo. Usually the doses of such medications are quite low, which may account for their continuing usefulness. A comparable situation probably exists in respect to caffeine. A substantial number of persons continue, day after day, to respond to a cup or two of coffee in the morning with a combination of psychological and physiological response. The same is true with drugs in these three classes, and even though part of the response may be psychological it does not lessen their usefulness.

In other patients, when one of these medications loses its effectiveness, another one may still produce a response. Even though there is usually some degree of cross-tolerance, switching from one preparation to another, especially if there are differences in chemical structure, may nonetheless enable the patient to continue medication in cases where it is indicated.

Justification for prolonged use is obvious when there is a primary indication but there are also instances when these drugs counteract the side effects of other necessary "major" medications and make such use possible when it would otherwise be unacceptable.

As with medications of all types, alternatives to long-term administration should be considered—psychotherapy, biofeedback, hypnosis, or even environmental manipulation if it is possible. If none of these are effective, the substitution of medications with a lower potential for abuse should be considered: low doses of major tranquilizers in place of minor tranquilizers or hypnotics (the risk of tardive dyskinesia is discussed in the preface); activating antidepressants instead of stimulants and drugs such as lithium, caffeine and L-tryptophan for selected use.

BIBLIOGRAPHY

1. Adams, H.B.: The influence of social variables, treatment methods, and administrative factors on mental hospital admission rates. *Psychiat. Quart.* 35 (1961):353–372.
2. Adelson, D., Epstein, L.J.: A study of phenothiazines with male and female chronically ill schizophrenic patients. *J. Ner. Ment. Dis.* 134 (1962):543,554.
3. Adler, A.: Office treatment of the chronic schizophrenic patient. *Proc. Amer. Psychopath. Ass.* 54 (1966):366–371.
4. Allert, M.-L., Schmitt, W.: Zur Fluphenazin-Therapie schizophrener Psychosen. *Pharmakopsychiat.* 2 (1969):66–74.
5. Alnaes, R., Kristiansen, J.: Desipramin (Sertofren) in the treatment of depression with a psychodynamic analysis of the therapeutic effect. 4th World Congr. Psychiat., Madrid 1966, Abstracts, Int. Congr. Ser. No. 117: p. 101; Excerpta Medica Foundation, Amsterdam 1966.
6. Angst, J.: Geschlecht, Intelligenz, praemorbide Persönlichkeit und Manifestationsalter in ihrer Bedeutung für Prognose und Verlauf endogen depressiver Psychosen. In: *Schizophrenie und Zyklothymie. Ergebnisse und Probleme*, hsg. von Huber, G., pp. 57–62; Thieme, Stuttgart 1969.
7. Angst, J., Baastrup, P., Grof, P., Schou, M., Weis, P.: Die Prophylaxe manisch-depressiv-schizophrener Mischpsychosen. In: *Neuroleptische Dauer- und Depottherapie in der Psychiatrie*, hsg. von Heinrich, K., pp. 106–112; Schnetztor-Verlag, Konstanz 1969.
8. Angst, J., Dittrich, A., Grof, P.: Course of endogenous affective psychoses and its modification by prophylactic administration of imipramine and lithium. *Int. Pharmacopsychiat.* 2 (1969):1–11.

8a. Angst, J., Frei, M., Beck, M., Jaenicke, U., Mueller, W., Padrutt, A., Scharfetter, C., Vetter, P., Zulauf, S.: Vergleich von Perphenazin (Trilafon-Tabletten) und Perphenazin-Oenanthat (Trilafon-Depot-Injektionen) im Doppelblindversuch. *Pharmakopsychiat.* 5 (1972), 169–176.

9. Angst, J., Grof, P., Hippius, H., Pöldinger, W., Weis, P.: La psychose maniaco-dépressive est-elle périodique ou intermittente? In: *Cycles biologiques et psychiatrie*, edit. Ajuriaguerra, J., pp. 339–351; Georg & Cie, Genève/Masson, Paris 1968.

10. Angst, J., Theobald, W.: Tofranil (Imipramine). Stämpfli & Cie AG, Berne 1970.

11. Angst, J., Weis, P.: Periodicity of depressive psychoses. V. Congress Collegium Internationale Neuro-Psychopharmacologicum, Washington, D.C., März 1966. Proc. Fifth, Int. Except. Med. Found. Int. Congr. Series No. 129 (1967):703–710; Elsevier, Amsterdam.

12. Angst, J., Weis, P., Grof, P., Baastrup, P.C., Schou, M.: Lithium prophylaxis in recurrent affective disorders. *Brit. J. Psychiat.* 116 (1970):604–614.

13. Anonymous: Evaluation of a new antipsychotic agent. Piperacetazine (Quide). *J. Amer. Med. Ass.* 215 (1971):783–784.

13a. Asperger, H.: Die autistischen Psychopathen in Kindesalter. *Arch. Psychiat.* Nervenkr. 117 (1944):7.

14. Authier, L., Tetreault, L., Vulpe, M., Kekhwa, G., Gagnon, M.A., Bordeleau, J.M.: L'association de Chlorpromazine et de Trifluoperazine: potentialisation et antagonisme de leurs effets antipsychotiques et extra-pyramidaux. *C.R. Congr. Psychiat. Neurol. Franç.* 66 (1968):455–466.

15. Ayd, F.J.: Neuroleptic-induced extrapyramidal reactions: incidence, manifestations and management. In: *The future of pharmacotherapy: new drug delivery systems*, edit. by Ayd, F.J., chapter 10, pp. 77–88; Int. Drug Therapy Newsletter, Baltimore 1973.

16. Ayd, F.J.: Perphenazine: a reappraisal after eight years. *Dis. Nerv. Syst.* 15 (1964):311–317.

17. Ayd, F.J.: Children born of mothers treated with chlorpromazine during pregnancy. *Clin. Med.* 71 (1964): 1758–1763.

18. Ayd, F.J.: Chlorpromazine: ten year's experience. In: *Neuropsychopharmacology*, edit. by Bradley, P.B., Flugel, F., Hoch, P.H., Vol. 3, pp. 572–574; Proceedings of the Third Meeting of the Collegium Internationale Neuropsychopharmacologicum; Elsevier, New York 1964.

19. Ayd, F.J.: Fluphenazine: twelve year's experience. *Dis. Nerv. Syst.* 29 (1968); 744–747.

20. Ayd, F.J.: Excretion of psychotropic drugs in human breast milk. *Int. Drug. Ther. Newsl.* 8 (1973): 33–40.
21. Baastrup, P.C.: The use of lithium in manic depressive psychoses. *Comprehens. Psychiat.* 5 (1964):396–408.
22. Baastrup, P.C., Poulsen, J.C., Schou, M., Thomsen, K., Amdisen, A.: Prophylactic lithium: double-blind discontinuation in manic-depressive and recurrent-depressive disorders. *Lancet* (1970/*ii*):326–330.
23. Baastrup, P.C., Schou, M.: Lithium as a prophylactic agent. Its effect against recurrent depressions and manic-depressive psychoses. *Arch. Gen. Psychiat.* 16 (1967):162–172.
24. Ballon, J.: Skin pigmentation and the phenothiazines. Electrocardiographic aspects. In: *Toxicity and adverse reactions studies with neuroleptics and antidepressants*, edit. by Lehmann, H.E., Ban, T.A., pp. 63–65; Quebec Psychopharmacological Research Ass., Verdun 1967.
25. Ballon, J.: Electrocardiographic changes with psychoactive drugs. The cardiologist's viewpoint. In: *Toxicity and adverse reaction studies with neuroleptics and antidepressants*, edit. by Lehmann, H.E., Ban, T.A., pp. 158–164.; Quebec Psychopharmacological Research Ass., Verdun 1967.
26. Baruk, H., Pécheny, J.: Essai clinique de l'imipramine 10mg en thérapeutique géronto-psychiatrique. *Annales Moreau de Tours*, Vol. 2, pp. 218–221; Presses Univ. France, Paris 1965.
27. Bauer, H., Girke, W., Kanowski, S., Krebs, F.A., Müller-Oerlinghausen, B.: Ergebnisse zum Problem der psychophysischen Ermüdung unter Lithium-Dauertherapie. *Activ. Nerv. Sup.* (Prag) 15 (1973):89–90.
28. Belfer, M.L., Shader, R.I.: Autonomic effects. In: *Psychotropic drug side effects*, edit. by Shader, R.I., DiMascio, A., pp. 116–123; Williams and Wilkins, Baltimore 1970.
29. Beumont, P.J.V., Corker, C.S., Friesen, H.G., Kolakowska, T., Mandelbrote, B.M., Marshall, J., Murray, M.A.F., Wiles, D.H.: The effects of phenothiazines on endocrine function: II. Effects in men and post-menopausal women. *Brit. J. Psychiat.* 124 (1974):420–430.
30. Beumont, P.J.V., Gelder, M.G., Friesen, H.G., Harris, G.W., MacKinnon, P.C.B., Mandelbrote, B.M., Wiles, D.H.: The effects of phenothiazines on endocrine function: I. Patients with inappropriate lactation and amenorrhoea. *Brit. J. Psychiat.* 124 (1974):413–419.

31. Bigelow, N., Ozerengin, F., Schneider, J., Sainz, A.: Carphenazine in the treatment of chronic schizophrenia. In: Cleghorn, R.A., Moll, A.E., Roberts, C.A.: *Third World Congress of Psychiatry Proceedings*, vol. 2, pp. 1102-1105, McGill University Press, Toronto 1962.

32. Bishop, M.P., Mason, L.B., Gallant, D.M.: Blood pressure abnormalities in schizophrenic patients: Some considerations relevant to the clinical testing of investigational drugs. *Curr. Ther. Res.* 10 (1968):315-322.

33. Bitnun, S.: Possible effects of clordiazepoxide on the fetus. *Canad. Med. Ass. J.* 100 (1969):351.

34. Blackwell, B., Shepherd, M.: Prophylactic lithium: another therapeutic myth? An examination of the evidence to date. *Lancet* (1968/*i*): 968-971.

35. Blair, J.H., Simpson, G.M.: Effect of antipsychotic drugs on reproductive functions. *Dis. Nerv. Syst.* 27 (1966):645-647.

36. Bleuler, M.: Endocrinological psychiatry and psychology. *Henry Ford Hosp. Med. J.* 15/4 (1967):309-317.

37. Bleuler, M.: Die schizophrenen Geistesstörungen im Licht langjähriger Kranken-und Familiengeschichten. Georg Thieme, Stuttgart 1972.

38. Bora, G.: Comparison of dosage ranges of carphenazine and trifluoperazine in elderly chronic schizophrenics. *Dis. Nerv. Syst.* 29 (1968):695-697.

39. Böszörmenyi, Z., Solti, G.: On the use of levomepromazine in psychiatry. *Ther. Hung.* 15 (1967):62-71.

40. Bourgeois, M.: Priapismes sous neuroleptiques (trois cas). *Nouv. Presse Méd.* 1 (1972):1161.

41. Buffa, P., Lacal, C.F., Lo Gullo, O., Pedretti, A., Armocide, C.C.: Sindrome depresivo involutivo y arterioscleroso. *Notas Ter.* 8 (1963):1-6.

42. Busfield, B.L., Schneller, P., Capra, D.: Depressive symptom or side effect? A comparative study of symptoms during pretreatment and treatment periods of patients on three antidepressant medications. *J. Nerv. Ment. Dis.* 134 (1962):339-345.

43. Cade, J.F.J.: Lithium salts in the treatment of psychotic excitement. *Med. J. Aust.* 36 (1949):349-352.

44. Carsoallen, H.B., Rochman, H., Lovergrove, T.D.: High dosage trifluoperazine in schizophrenia. *Canad. Psychiat. Ass. J.* 13 (1968):459-461.

45. Colmart, C., Bridgman, F., Girard, B.: La thiopropérazine et la lévomépromazine utilisées en association dans le traitement des psychoses chroniques. *Evolut. Psychiat.* 34 (1969):849-860.

46. Coppen, A.: Paper read at IGSAD Meeting. Varenna 1975 (unpublished).
47. Coppen, A., Noguera, R., Bailey, J., Burns, B.H., Swani, M.S., Hare, E.H., Gardner, R., Maggs, R.,: Prophylactic lithium in affective disorders. (Controlled trial). *Lancet* (1971/*ii*):275–279.
48. Cowley, L.M.: Evaluation of Carphenazine in hospitalized schizophrenic women. *Dis. Nerv. Syst.* 28 (1967):126–130.
49. Cundall, R.L., Brooks, P.W., Murray, L.G.: A controlled evaluation of lithium prophylaxis in affective disorders. *Psychol. Med.* 2 (1972):308–311.
50. Curran, J.P.: Management of tardive dyskinesia with thiopropazate. *Amer. J. Psychiat.* 130 (1973):925–927.
51. Dardenne, M.U.: Ist Kaffee bei Glaukom erlaubt? *Med. Klin.* 62 (1967):858.
51a. Davis, J., Clyman, M.J., Decker, A., Bronstein, S., Roland, M.: Effect of phenelzine on semen in infertility: A preliminary report. *Fertil. Steril.* 17 (1966):221–225.
52. Deberdt, R.: De l'intérêt des associations neuroleptiques incisifs-neuroleptiques sédatifs: notre expérience pendant huit ans de l'association Thiopropérazine-Lévomépromazine. *C.R. Congr. Psychiat. Neurol. Franç.* 66 (1968):477–483.
53. Delay, J., Deniker, P., Harl, J.M.: Utilisation en thérapeutique psychiatrique d'une phénothiazine d'action centrale élective (4560 R.P.) *Ann. Méd.-Psychol.* 110 (1952):112.
54. Dengler, K.: Beitrag zur Infusionstherapie mit Fluphenazin bei Schizophrenen im Hinblick auf die Steuerbarkeit der neuroleptischen Schwelle. *Med. Welt* 20 (1969):977–981.
55. Desmond, M.M., Rudolph, A.J., Hill, R.M., Claghorn, J.L., Dreessen, P.R., Burgdorff, I.: Behavioral alterations in infants born to mothers on psychoactive medication during pregnancy. *Tex. Inst. Mental Sci.* Nov. 1968:20–23.
56. Dinity, S., Scarpitti, F.R., Albini, J.L., Lefton, M., Pasamanick, B.: An experimental study in the prevention of hospitalization of schizophrenics. *Amer. J. Orthopsychiat.* 35 (1965):1–9.
57. Dynes, J.B.: Sudden death. *Dis. Nerv. Syst.* 30 (1969):24–28.
58. Ebert, M.H., Shader, R.I.: Cardiovascular effects. In: *Psychotropic drug side effects*, edit. by Shader, R.I., DiMascio, A., pp.149–163; Williams and Wilkins, Baltimore 1970.
59. Ebert, M.H., Shader, R.I.: Hematological effects. In: *Psychotropic drug side effects*, edit. by Shader, R.I., DiMascio, A., 164–174; Williams and Wilkins, Baltimore 1970.

60. Edler, K., Gottfries, C.G., Haslund, J., Ravn, J.: Eye changes in connection with neuroleptic treatment especially concerning phenothiazines and thioxanthenes. *Acta Psychiat. Scand.* 47 (1971):377–385.

61. Efendiyeva, D.G.: Use of nozinan in psychiatric practice. In *Voprosy Psikhofarmakologii*, edit by Rokhlin, L.L., Avrutskiy, G.Ya., 8532–551; USSR Ministry of Public Health, Moscow 1967.

62. Eggermont, E.,: Withdrawal symptoms in neonates associated with maternal imipramine therapy. *Lancet* (1973/*ii*):680.

63. Eggermont, E., Raveschot, J., Deneve, V., Casteels van Daele, M.: The adverse influence of imipramine of the adaption of the newborn infant to extrauterine life. *Acta Paediat. Belg.* 26 (1972):197–204.

64. Elie,, R., Morin, L., Tetreault, L.: Effets de l'Ethopropazine et du Trihexyphénidyle sur quelques paramètres du syndrome neuroleptique. *Encéphale* 61 (1972):32–52.

65. Emerson, C.H., Dyson, W.L., Utiger, R.D.: Serum thyrotropin and thyroxine concentrations in patients receiving lithium carbonate. *J. Clin. Endocr.* 36 (1973), 338–346.

66. Engelhardt, D.M., Freedman, N.: Maintenance drug therapy: The schizophrenic patient in the community. In: *Psychopharmocology*, edit. by Kline, N.S., Lehmann, H.E., pp. 933–960; Little Brown & Co., Boston 1965.

67. Engelhardt, D.M., Freedman, M., Hankoff, L.D., Mann, D., Margolis, R.: Long-term drug-induced symptom modification in schizophrenic outpatients. *J. Nerv. Ment. Dis.* 137 (1963):231–241.

68. Engelhardt, D.M., Rosen, B., Freedman, N., Mann, D., Margolis, R.: Phenothiazines in prevention of psychiatric hospitalization. II. Duration of treatment exposure. *J. Amer. Med. Ass.* 186 (1963):981–983.

69. Eveloff, H.H.: Pediatric psychopharmacology. In: *Principles of psychopharmacology: a textbook for physicians, medical students and behavioral scientists*, edit. by Clark, W.D., del Giudice, J., pp. 683–694; Academic Press, New York 1970.

70. Fann, W.E., Davis, J.M., Wilson, I.C.: Methylphenidate in tardive dyskinesia. *Amer. J. Psychiat.* 130 (1973), 922–924.

71. Ferguson, J.: The disadvantage of a maintenance dose of neuroplegics for patients returned to society. *Psychiat. Neurol. Neurochir.* 64 (1961):267–276.

72. Flowers, C.E., Rudolph, A.J., Desmond, M.M.: Diazepam (Valium) as an adjunct in obstetric analgesia. *Obstet. Gynec.* 34 (1969):68–81.

73. Forrest, F.M., Snow, H.L.: Prognosis of eye complications caused by phenothiazines. *Dis. Nerv. Syst.* 29, Suppl.3 (1968):26–28.

74. Forrest, F.M., Snow, H.L., Erickson, G., Geiter, C.W., Laxson, G.O.: Incidence of late "Melanosis" side effects in chronic mental patients after long term phenothiazine therapy. *Proc. W. Pharmacol. Soc.* 9 (1966):18–20.

75. Gallant, D.M., Bishop, M.P.: Quide and mellaril in chronic schizophrenic patients. *Curr. Ther. Res.* 14 (1972):10–16.

76. Gallant, D.M., Edwards, C.G., Bishop, M.P., Galbraith, G.C.: Withdrawal symptoms after abrupt cessation of antipsychotic compounds: Clinical confirmation in chronic schizophrenics. *Amer. J. Psychiat.* 121 (1964):491–493.

77. Gantz, R.S., Birkett, D.P.: Phenothiazine reduction as a course of rehospitalization. *Arch. Gen. Psychiat.* 12 (1965):586–588.

78. Gelina, L.I., Golovan, L.I., Kogan, A.D.: Opyt premeneniya neyleptila v praktike detskoy psikhiatrii. *Z. Nevropat. Psihiat.* 67 (1967):906–911.

79. Gessa, R. et al.: Blockade by apomorphine of haloperidol-induced dyskinesia in schizophrenic patients. *Lancet* (1972/*ii*):981.

80. Greiner, A.C.: Schizophrenia melanosis. Iatrogenic-congenital defect. *Dis. Nerv. Syst.* 29, Suppl. 3 (1968):14–15.

81. Greiner, A.C.: Phenothiazines and diffuse melanosis. *Agressologie* 9 (1968):219–224.

82. Grof, P., Vinar, O.: Maintenance and prophylactic imipramine doses in recurrent depressions. *Activ. Nerv. Sup.* (Praha) 8 (1966):383–385.

83. Gross, G., Huber, G., Schüttler, R.: Verlaufsuntersuchungen bei Schizophrenen. In: *2. Weissenauer schizophrenie-symposion, 4.+5.* Mai 1973, hsg. von Huber, G., pp. 101–118; F.K.Schattauer Verlag, Stuttgart-New York 1973.

84. Gunn, D.R.: Skin pigmentation and the phenothiazine. A psychiatrist's comments. In: *Toxicity and adverse reaction studies with neuroleptics and antidepressants*, edit by Lehmann, H.E., Ban, T.A., pp. 72–74; Quebec Psychopharmacological Research Association, Verdun 1967.

85. Haase, H.J.: Therapie mit Psychopharmaka und anderen psychotropen Medikamenten, F.K.Schattauer, Stuttgart 1972.

86. Hamilton, M.: Therapeutic effects of phenelzine. Collegium Internationale Neuropsychopharmacologicum, IX. Congr., Paris, 7–12.7.1974; symposia, abstracts in: *J. Pharmacol.* 5 / Suppl.1 (1974):102.

87. Hamon, J. Paraire, J. Velluz, J.: Remarques sur l'action du 4560 R.P. sur l'agitation maniaque. *Ann. Méd.-Psychol.* 110 (1952):331.

88. Hanesson, I.: Carphenazine in the intensive care of chronically ill psychotics. *Int. J. Neuropsychiat.* 3 (1967):332-336.

89. Harrer, G.: Zur Inkompatibilität zwischen Monoaminooxydase-Hemmern und Imipramin. *Wien. Med. Wschr.* 111 (1961):551-553.

90. Harrer, G.: Inkompatibilitätserscheinungen bei Psychopharmaka. Neuro-Psycho-Pharmacology, Proc. 5th Meet. C.I.N.P., Washington 1966. Int. Congr. Ser. No. 129, pp. 588-594 (Excerpta Medica Foundation, Amsterdam 1967).

91. Hartigan, G.P.: Paper read to the Southern Branch of the Royal Medico-Psychological Society. 1959 (unpublished).

92. Heinrich, K.: Zur Bedeutung des postremissiven Erschöpfungs-Syndroms für die Rehabilitation Schizophrener. *Nervenarzt* 38 (1967):487-491.

93. Heinrich, K.: Zur Aetiologie des postremissiven Erschöpfungs-Syndroms bei Schizophrenen. In *Pharmakopsychiatrische probleme in klinik und praxis*, hsg. von Heinrich, K., pp. 47-59; F.K.Schattauer Verlag, Stuttgart 1969.

94. Helmchen, H., Hippius, H.: Erscheinungsweise depressiver Syndrome unter der Therapie mit Neuroleptika. In *Pharmakopsychiatrische probleme in klinik und praxis*, hsg. von Heinrich, K. pp. 61-67; F.K.Schattauer Verlag, Stuttgart 1969.

95. Hershon, H.I., Kennedy, P.F., McGuire, R.J.: Persistence of extrapyramidal disorders and psychiatric relapse after withdrawal of long-term phenothiazine therapy. *Brit. J. Psychiat.* 120 (1972):41-50.

96. Hertz, D., Sulman, F.G.: Preventing depression with tryptophan. *Lancet* (1968/i):531-532.

97. Hill, R.M., Desmond, M.M., Kay, J.L.: Extrapyramidal dysfunction in an infant of a schizophrenic mother. *J. Pediat.* 69 (1966):589-595.

98. Hippius, H.: Zur Strukturanalyse der Wirkung von Psychopharmaka bei Schizophrenen. *Angl. Germ. Med. Rev.* 2 (1965):634-645.

99. Hippius, H.: Die Rolle der Psychopharmaka in der Psychiatrie der Gemeinschaft. In Lopez Ibor, J.J.: *Weltkongress für psychiatrie*, Internat. Congr. Series 117, p. 16. Excerpta Medica Foundation, Amsterdam 1966.

100. Hogarty, G., Goldberg, S.C.: Drug and social therapy in schizophrenic outpatients. *Psychopharm. Bull.* 8 (1972):18.

101. Holden, J.M.C., Holden, U.P.: Weight changes with schizophrenic psychosis and psychotropic drug therapy. *Psychosomatics* 11 (1970):551-561.

102. Holden, J.M.C., Itil, T.M.: Laboratory changes with chlordiazepoxide and thioridazine, alone and combined. *Canad. Psychiat. Ass. J.* 14 (1969):299–301.
103. Hollister, L.E., Hall, R.A.: Phenothiazine derivatives and morphologic changes in the liver. *Amer. J. Psychiat.* 123 (1966):211–212.
104. Honigfeld, G., Rosenblum, M.P., Blumenthal, J.I., Lambert, H.L., Roberts, A.J.: Behavioral improvement in the older schizophrenic patient: Drug and social therapies. *J. Amer. Geriat. Soc.* 13 (1965):57–72.
105. Hrushka, M., Bruck, M., Hsu, J.: Therapeutic effects of different modes of chlorpromazine administration. *Dis. Nerv. Syst.* 27 (1966):522–527.
105a. Hsu, J.J., Yap, A.T.: Autonomic reactions in relation to psychotropic drugs. *Dis. Nerv. Syst.* 28 (1967):304–310.
106. Hullin, R.P., McDonald, R., Allsopp, M.N.E.: Prophylactic lithium in recurrent affective disorders. *Lancet* (1972/*i*):1044–1046.
107. Hussain, M.Z., Khan, A.G., Chaudhry, Z.A.: Aplastic anemia associated with lithium therapy. *Canad. Med. Ass. J.* 108 (1973):724–728.
108. Imlah, N.W., Murphy, K.P.: The clinical use of longacting psychotropic drugs. *Psycopharmacologia (Berl.)* 26, Suppl. (1972):105.
109. Itil, T.M., Keskiner, A.: Fluphenazine hydrochloride, enenthate, and decanoate in the management of chronic psychosis. *Dis. Nerv. Syst.* 31, Suppl. 9 (1970):37–42.
110. Johnstone, E.C., Marsh, W.: The relationship between acetylator status and response to the monoamine oxydase inhibitor drug, phenelzine, in depressed patients. IX C.I.N.P. Congress: present status in research and clinical use of MAO-inhibitors; July 7–12, 1974, Paris; *J. Pharmacol.* 5/suppl.1 (1974):101.
111. Jokinen, A.-L.: Drug therapy for psychiatric outpatients. In: Lopez Ibor, J.J.: *Weltkongress für psychiatrie.* Internat. Congr. Series 117, pp. 243–244, Excerpta Medica Foundation, Amsterdam 1966.
112. Jung, E.G., Schwarz-Speck, M., Kormany, G.: Beitrag zur Photoallergie auf Chlorphenothiazine. *Schweiz. Med. Wschr.* 93 (1963):249–250.
112a. Kanner, L.: Autistic disturbances of affective contact. *Nerv. Child* 2 (1943):217.
113. Kay, D.W.K., Fahy, T., Garside, R.F.: A seven-month double-blind trial of amitriptyline and diazepam in ECT-treated depressed patients. *Brit. J. Psychiat.* 117 (1970):667–671.
114. Kazamatsuri, H., Chien, C.-P., Cole, J.O.: Treatment of tardive dyskinesia. I. Clinical efficacy of a dopamine-depleting agent, tetrabenazine.*Arch. Gen. Psychiat.* 27 (1972):95–103.

115. Kimbrough, J.C.: Incontinence with doxepine. *J. Amer. Med. Ass.* 221 (1972):510.

116. Klawans, H.L., Rubovits, R.: An experimental model of tardive dyskinesia. *J. Neural. Transm.* 33 (1972):235–246.

117. Kline, N.S.: The future of drugs and drugs of the future. *J. Soc. Issues* 27 (1971):73–87.

118. Kline, N.S.: Manipulation of life patterns with drugs. In: *Psychotropic drugs in the year 2000: use by normal humans*, edit. by Evans, W.O., Kline, N.S., chapter 6, pp. 69–85; Charles C Thomas, Springfield, Ill.

119. Kline, N.S.: A narrative account of lithium usage in psychiatry. In: *Lithium: its role in psychiatric research and treatment*, edit. by Gershon, S., Shopsin, B., chapter 1, pp. 5–13; Plenum Publ.Co., New York 1973.

120. Kline, N.S., Brill, H.: A plan and a detailed budget for an evaluation of the new drugs. In: *Psychopharmacology*, edit. by Cole, J.O., Gerard, R.W.:447–453; National Academy of Sciences–National Research Council Publ. 583, Washington 1959.

121. Korczyn, A.D.: Pathophysiology of drug induced dyskinesias. *Neuropharmacology* 11 (1972):601–607.

122. Korenyi, C., Lowenstein, B.: Chlorpromazine induced diabetes. *Dis. Nerv. Syst.* 29 (1968):827–828.

123. Kozakova, M.: Drug purpura after antidepressive drugs (tschech.) *Cls. Derm.* 46 (1971):158–160.

124. Kris, E.B.: Aftercare and rehabilitation of the mentally ill. *Curr. Ther. Res.* 5 (1963):24–30.

125. Kuznetsov, O.N.: Primeneniye etaperazine u bolnykh paranoidnoy formoy shizofrenii. In: *Voprosy Psikhofarmakologii,* edit. by Rokhlin, L.L., Avrutskiy, G.Ya., 192–201; USSR Ministry of Public Health, Moscow 1967.

126. Laborit, H., Hugenard, P.: L'hibernation artificielle par moyens pharmaco-dynamiques et physiques. *Press Méd.* 59 (1951):1329.

127. Lader, M.H.: Prophylactic lithium? *Lancet* (1968/*ii*):103.

127a. Landolt, H.: *Die Temporallappenepilepsie und ihre Psychopathologie.* Karger, Basel-New York 1960.

128. Lauber, H.: Studie zur Frage der Krankheitsdauer unter Behandlung mit Psychopharmaka. *Nervenarzt* 35 (1964):488–491.

129. Lazos, G., Kapetanakis, S., Photiades, H.: Lactation in male mammary glands after treatment with psychotropic drugs. Immunoelectrophoretic study of the secretion. (Greek) *Acta Neurol. Psychiat. Hellen.* 11 (1972):154–163.

130. Lee, H., Lehmann, H.E., Ban, T.A.: Skin pigmentation and the phenothiazine. Clinical aspects. In: *Toxicity and adverse reaction studies with neuroleptics and antidepressants*, edit. by Lehmann, H.E., Ban, T.A., 75–78; Quebec Psychopharmacological Research Association, Verdun 1967.

131. Leuenberger, A., Labhardt, F.: Psychopharmaka und Glaukom. *Ther. Umsch.* 12 (1965:184–185.

132. Lien, J.B.: Thioproperazine ("Majeptil"), therapeutic results and complications in sixty-three patients with functional psychoses. *Acta Psychiat. Scand.* 43 (1967):318–340.

133. Linden, K.J., Knaack, M., Edel, W.: Die Kombination von rating scales und Handschrifttests zur Objektivierung und Quantifizierung neuroleptischer Effekte. Eine Doppelblindstudie mit Fluspirilene und Penfluridol. In: *Psychopharmocology, sexual disorders and drug abuse*. Proceedings of the Symposia held at the VIII Congress of the Collegium Internationale Neuro-Psychopharmacologicum, Copenhagen 1972; edit. by Ban, T.A. et al., 273–278; North-Holland Publishing Company, Amsterdam-London 1973.

134. Lochner, K.H., Scheuing, M.R., Flach, F.F.: The effect of 1-triiod-thyronine on chronic schizophrenic patients. *Acta Psychiat. Scand.* 39 (1963): 413–426.

135. De Long, S.L.: Incidence and significance of chlorpromazine induced eye changes. *Dis. Nerv. Syst.* 29, Suppl.3 (1968):19–22.

136. Lovett-Doust, J.W., Huszka, L.: Influence of some psychoactive drugs on mineral metabolism in man. *Int. Pharmacopsychiat.* 8 (1973): 159–172.

137. Lüllmann, H., Lüllmann-Rauch, R., Wassermann, O.: Arneimittel-induzierte Phospholipidspeicherkrankheit. *Dtsch. Med. Wschr.* 98 (1973): 1616–1625.

138. Makela, S.: Perfenazin som aktiverande fentiazin. *Nord. Psykiat. T.* 20 (1966):208–220.

139. Mann, A.M., Macpherson, A.S.: Clinical experience with imipramine (G 22355) in the treatment of depression. *Canad. Psychiat. Ass. J.* 4 (1959):38–47.

140. Margat, M.-P., Broussot, T.: Application du chlorhydrate de Flu-phénazine, relavé par l'OEnanthate de Fluphénazine, chez 40 schizophrènes et délirants chroniques. *C.R. Congr. Psychiat. Neurol. Franç.* 66 (1968):602–606.

141. Marjerrison, G., Irvine, D., Stewart, C.N., Williams, R., Matheu, H., Demay, M.: Withdrawal of long-term phenothiazines from chronically hospitalized psychiatric patients. *Canad. Psychiat. Ass. J.* 90 (1964):290–298.

142. Marks, J.: Interactions involving drugs used in psychiatry. Scientific basis of drug therapy in psychiatry, Symp. London 1964, pp. 191–201; Pergamon Press, Oxford 1965.

143. Mastrogiovanni, P.D.: Tofranil in gerontopsichiatria. *Rass. Neuropsychiat.* 18 (1964):107–121.

144. Matsuki, A., Oyama, T., Izai, S., Zsigmond, E.K.: Excessive mortality in schizophrenic patients on chronic phenothiazine treatment. *Agressologie* 13 (1972):407–418.

145. McAndrew, J.B., Case, O., Treffert, D.A.: Effects of prolonged phenothiazine intake on psychotic and other hospitalized children. *J. Autism. Childh. Schiz.* 2 (1972):75–91.

146. Meier-Ewert, K., Baumgart, H.-H., Friedenberg, P.: Thromboembolische Komplikationen bei neuro- und thymoleptischer Behandlung. *Dtsch. Med. Wschr.* 92 (1967):2174–2178.

147. Melia, P.I.: Prophylactic lithium: A double-blind trial in recurrent affective disorders. *Brit. J. Psychiat.* 116 (1970):621–624.

148. Merrill, D.C., Markland, C.: Vesical dysfunction induced by the major tranquilizers. *J. Urol.* (Baltimore) 107 (1972):769–776.

149. Meusert, W.: Die Behandlung endogen-depressiver Verstimmungszustände in der psychiatrischen Praxis. *Medizinische* (1959):2582–2585.

150. Mindham, R.H.S., Howland, C., Shepherd, M.: An evaluation of continuation therapy with tricyclic antidepressants in depressive illness. *Psychol. Med.* 3 (1973):5–17.

151. Moir, D.C., Dingwall-Fordyce, I., Weir, R.D.: Medicines evaluation and monitoring group. A follow-up study of cardiac patients receiving amitriptyline. *Europ. J. Clin. Pharmacol.* 6 (1973):98–101.

152. Montero, E.: Thioridazine compared with a combination of chlorpromazine and trifluoperazine hydrochloride in schizophrenic patients. V. World Congress of Psychiatry, Abstracts, Prensa Médica Mexicana 1971 (Nr.878).

153. Moore, M.T., Book, M.H.: Sudden death in phenothiazine therapy. A clinico-pathologic study of twelve cases. *Psychiat. Quart.* 44 (1970):389–402.

154. Morton, M.R.: A study of the withdrawal of chlorpromazine or trifluoperazine in chronic schizophrenia. *Amer. J. Psychiat.* 124 (1967):1585–1588.

155. Nemeth, J., Petrovich, M.: Chlorpromazine and trifluoperazine treatment. *Dis. Nerv. Syst.* 28 (1967):812–814.

156. Nies, A., Robinson, D.S., Ravaris, C.L., Ives, J.O.: The efficacy of the MAO-inhibitor phenelzine: dose effects and prediction of response. Collegium Internationale Neuropsychopharmacologi-

cum, IX. congr., Paris, 7.–12.7.1974; symposia, abstracts in: *J. Pharmacol.* 5 / suppl. 1 (1974):100–101.

157. Novak, E.N.: The effect of chlorpromazine on the blood coagulation (Russian). *Farmakol.i Toksikol.* 35 (1972):717–720.

158. Orlov, P., Kasparian, G., DiMascio, A., Cole, J.O.: Withdrawal of anti-parkinson drugs. *Arch. Gen. Psychiat.* 25 (1971):410–412.

159. Overall, J.E., Hollister, L.E., Honigfeld, G., Kimbell, I.H., Jr., Meyer, F., Bennett, J.L., Caffey, E., Jr.: Comparison of acetophenazine with perphenazine in schizophrenics; demonstration of differential effects based on computer-derived diagnostic models. *Clin. Pharmacol. Ther.* 4 (1963):200–208.

160. Panzetta, A.F.: Toward a scientific psychiatric nosology. conceptual and pragmatic issues. *Arch. Gen. Psychiat.* 30 (1974):154–161.

161. Paulson, G.W.: An evaluation of the permanence of the "tardive dyskinesias". *Dis. Nerv. Syst.* 29 (1968):692–694.

162. Peele, R., von Loetzen, I.S.: Phenothiazine deaths: a critical review. *Amer. J. Psychiat.* 130 (1973):306–309.

163. Pfeiffer, W.M.: Klinisch-therapeutische Erfahrungen mit Fluphenazin. *Arzneimittel-Forsch.* 17 (1967):1327–1329.

164. Pisciotta, A.V.: Studies on agranulocytosis. IX. A biochemical defect in chlorpromazine sensitive marrow cells. *J. Lab. Clin. Med.* 78 (1971):435–448.

165. Platz, A.R., Klett, C.J., Caffey, E.M., Jr.: Selective drug action related to chronic schizophrenic subtype: a comparative study of carphenazine, chlorpromazine and trifluoperazine. *Dis. Nerv. Syst.* 28 (1967):601–605.

166. Polizos, P., Engelhardt, D.M., Hoffman, S.P., Waizer, J.: Neurological consequences of psychotropic drug withdrawal in schizophrenic children. *J. Autism. Childh. Schiz.* 3 (1973):247–253.

167. Pöldinger, W.: Kompendium der Psychopharmakotherapie. Wissenschaftlicher Dienst Roche, Basel 1971.

168. Praag, H.M.van., Schut, T., Dols, L., Schilfgaarden, R.van.: Controlled trial of penfluridol in acute psychosis. *Brit. Med. J.* 4 (1971):710–713.

169. Prien, R.F.: Prophylactic treatment of recurrent depression: observations from a multihospital collaborative study. In: *Classification and prediction of outcome of depression*, edit. by Angst, J., pp. 117–127; F.K. Schattauer Verlag, Stuttgart–New York 1974.

170. Prien, R.F., Caffey, E.M., Jr., Klett, C.J.: Prophylactic efficacy of lithium carbonate in manic-depressive illness. Report of the Veterans Administration and National Institute of Mental Health collaborative study group. *Arch. Gen. Psychiat.* 28 (1973):337–341.

171. Prien, R.F., Cole, J.O.: High dose chlorpromazine therapy in chronic schizophrenia. Report of National Institute of Mental Health—Psychopharmacology research branch collaborative study group. *Arch. Gen. Psychiat.* 18 (1968):482–495.

172. Prien, R.F., Cole, J.O., Belkin, N.F.: Relapse in chronic schizophrenics following abrupt withdrawal of tranquilizing medication. *Brit. J. Psychiat.* 115 (1969), 679–686.

173. Prien, R.F., Klett, C.J., Caffey, E.M., Jr.: Lithium carbonate and imipramine in prevention of affective episodes. A comparison in recurrent affective illness. Report of the Veterans Administration and National Institute of Mental Health collaborative study group, Washington. *Arch. Gen. Psychiat.* 29 (1973):420–425.

174. Prien, R.F., Klett, C.J., Caffey, E.M., Jr.: Lithium prophylaxis in recurrent affective illness. *Amer. J. Psychiat.* 131 (1974):198–203.

175. Prien, R.F., Levine, J., Cole, J.O.: High dose trifluoperazine therapy in chronic schizophrenia. *Amer. J. Psychiat.* 126 (1969):305–313.

176. Prien, R.F., Levine, J., Cole, J.O.: Indications for high dose chlorpromazine therapy in chronic schizophrenia. *Dis. Nerv. Syst.* 31 (1970):739–745.

177. Rajotte, P., Denber, H.C.B.: Long-term community follow up of formerly hospitalized psychotic patients. *J. Nerv. Ment. Dis.* 136 (1963):445–454.

178. Reznikoff, L.: Imipramine therapy of depressive syndromes. *Amer. J. Psychiat.* 116 (1960):1110–1111.

179. Richardson, H.: The historical approach to the theory of diagnosis. *Brit. J. Psychiat.* 122 (1973):245–250.

180. Richter, H.-E.: Soziale Aspekte der ambulanten Dauertherapie mit Psychopharmaka. *Dtsch. Med. J.* 12 (1961):532–533.

181. Roberts, F.J.: Single daily dose treatment of psychiatric patients with phenothiazine derivatives. *J. Ment. Sci.* 107 (1961):104–108.

182. Rona, G.: Skin pigmentation and the phenothiazines. Histogenesis. In: *Toxicity and adverse reaction studies with neuroleptics and antidepressants*, edit. by Lehmann, H.E., Ban, T.A., pp. 97–99; Quebec Psychopharm. Res. Ass., Verdun 1967.

183. Rona, G.: Electrocardiographic changes with psychoactive drugs. The pathologist's viewpoint. In: *Toxicity and adverse reaction studies with neuroleptics and antidepressants*, edit. by Lehmann, H.E., Ban, T.A., pp. 165–167; Quebec Psychopharm. Res. Ass., Verdun 1967.

184. Ropert, P.: Technique et place de la cure neuroleptique par perphénazine en psychiatrie. *Psychopharmacologie:* Suppl. Encéphale, Mars–Avril (1971):71–82.

185. Rysanek, K., Konig, J., Spankova, H., Mlejnkova, M.: Effect of tricyclic antidepressants on phosphodiesterase. Correlation between aggregability and thrombocyte metabolism. *Activ. Nerv. Sup.* (Prag) 15 (1973):126–127.

186. Sabouraud, O., LeBorgne, Y.-R., Assicot, P., Bourel, J.: Intérêt d'une nouvelle forme médicamenteuse associant un neuroleptique et ses correcteurs. *C.R. Congr. Psychiat. Neurol. Franç.* 67 (1969):707–712.

187. Safer, D.J., Allen, R.P.: Factors influencing the suppressant effects of two stimulant drugs on the growth of hyperactive children. *Pediatrics* 51 (1973):660–667.

188. Sainz, A.: Antipsychotic spectrum of proketazine. *Dis. Nerv. Syst.* 22 (1961):585–587.

189. Sainz, A.:Comparison of the clinical effects of carphenazine and fluphenazine in chronic schizophrenics. *Dis. Nerv. Syst.* 22 (1961): 77–79.

190. Sainz, A., Ozerengin, F., Sanchez, N., Ferreri, V.J.: The phrenopraxic spectrum of acetophenazine. *Dis. Nerv. Syst.* 23 (1962):714–717.

191. Saldanha, V.F., Havard, C.W.H., Bird, R., Gardner, R.: The effect of chlorpromazine on pituitary function. *Clin. Endocr.* (Oxford) 1 (1972):173–180.

192. Saran, B.M.: Lithium. *Lancet* (1969/*i*):1208–1209.

193. Schooler, N.R., Boothe, H.: Life history and length of hospital stay in schizophrenia. *Psychopharm. Bull.* 8 (1972): 17–18.

194. Schou, M.: Heutiger Stand der Lithium-Rezidivprophylaxe bei endogenen affektiven Erkrankungen. *Nervenarzt* 45 (1974):397–418.

195. Schou, M., Goldfield, M.D., Weinstein, M.R., Villeneuve, A.: Lithium and pregnancy. I. Report from the register of lithium babies. *Brit. Med. J.* (*1973*/21.April):135–136.

196. Schou, M., Amdisen, A., Steenstrup, O.R.: Lithium and pregnancy. II. Hazards to women given lithium during pregnancy and delivery. *Brit. Med. J.* (*1973*/21.April):137.

197. Schou, M., Amdisen, A.: Lithium and pregnancy. III. Lithium ingestion by children breast-fed by women on lithium treatment. *Brit. Med. J.* (*1973*/21.April):138.

198. Schou, M., Thomsen, K., Baastrup, P.C.: Studies on the course of recurrent endogenous affective disorders. *Int. Pharmacopsychiat.* 5 (1970):100–106.

199. Schou, M., Thomsen, K.: Lithium prophylaxis of recurrent endogenous affective disorders. In: *Lithium research and therapy,* edit. by Johnson, F.N., pp. 63–84; Academic Press, London-New York-San Francisco 1975.

200. Semenovskaya, E.I.: Affektivnyye narusheniya pri lechenii neyrolep-
tikami detey i podrostkov, stradayushchickh shizofreniyey. Z.
Nevropat. Psihiat. 67 (1967):1529–1534.
201. Shader, R.I.: Male sexual function. In: Psychotropic drug side effects,
edit. by Shader, R.I., DiMascio, A., pp. 63–71; Williams & Wilkins,
Baltimore 1970.
202. Shader, R.I.: Ejaculation disorders. In: Psychotropic drug side effects,
edit. by Shader, R.I., DiMascio, A., pp. 72–76; Williams & Wilkins,
Baltimore 1970.
203. Shader, R.I.: Pregnancy and psychotropic drugs. In: Psychotropic
drug side effects, edit. by Shader, R.I., DiMascio, A., pp. 206–213;
Williams & Wilkins, Baltimore 1970.
204. Shader, R.I.: Sexual dysfunction associated with mesoridazine besylate
(Serentil). Psychopharmacologia (Berl.) 27 (1972):293–294.
205. Shader, R.I., Belfer, M.L., DiMascio, A.: Thyroid function. In:
Psychotropic drug side effects, edit. by Shader, R.I., DiMascio, A.,
pp. 25–45; Williams & Wilkins, Baltimore 1970.
206. Shader, R.I., Belfer, M.L., DiMascio, A.: Glucose metabolism. In:
Psychotropic drug side effects, edit. by Shader, R.I., DiMascio, A.,
46–62; Williams & Wilkins, Baltimore 1970.
207. Shader, R.I., DiMascio, A.: Galactorrhea and gynecomastia. In:
Psychotropic drug side effects, edit. by Shader, R.I., DiMascio, A.,
4–9; Williams & Wilkins, Baltimore 1970.
207a. Shader, R.I., Giller, D.R., DiMascio, A.: Hypothalamic-pituitary-
adrenal axis. In: Psychotropic drug side effects, edit. by Shader,
R.I., DiMascio, A., pp. 16–24; Williams & Wilkins, Baltimore 1970.
208. Sherlock, S.: Jaundice due to drugs and poisons. In: Diseases of the
liver and biliary system, pp. 293–313; Blackwell, Oxford 1963.
209. Shopsin, B., Kline, N.S.: Combined tricyclic and monoamine oxidase
inhibitor (MAOI) therapy in depressed outpatients. Collegium
Internationale Neuropsychopharmacologicum, IX. Congr., Paris,
7.–12.7.1974; symposia, abstracts in: J. Pharmacol. 5 /suppl. 1
(1974):103.
210. Shopsin, B., Shenkman, L., Blum, M., Hollander, C.S.: Iodine and
lithium induced hypothyroidism. Documentation of synergism.
Amer. J. Med. 55 (1973):695–699.
211. Simonson, M.: Phenothiazine depressive reaction. Amer. J. Psychiat.
124 (1967):108.
212. Simpson, G.M.: Long-acting, antipsychotic agents and extrapyramidal
side effects. Dis. Nerv. Syst. 31, Suppl. 9 (1970):12–14.
213. Simpson, G.M., Amin, M., Kunz-Bartholini, E., Salim, T., Watts,
T.P.S.: Problems in the evaluation of the optimal dose of a butyro-

phenone (trifluperidol). *Internat. Pharmacopsychiat.* 2 (1969):59–70.

214. Simpson, G.M., Amin, M., Kunz-Bartholini, E., Watts, T.P.S., Laska, E.: Problems in the evaluation of the optimal dose of a phenothiazine (Butaperazine). *Dis. Nerv. Syst.* 29 (1968):478–484.

215. Simpson, G.M., Angus, J.W.S.: A preliminary study of prothipendyl in chronic schizophrenia. *Curr. Ther. Res.* 9 (1967):265–268.

216. Simpson, R.C.: Depression and imipramine. *Lancet* (1960/*i*):498.

217. Singh, M.M., Vergel de Dios, L., Kline, N.S.: Weight as a correlate of clinical response to psychotropic drugs. *Psychosomatics* 11 (1970): 562–570.

218. Snyder, S.H., Taylor, K.M., Coyle, J.T., Meyerhoff, J.L.: The role of brain dopamine in behavioral regulation and the actions of psychotropic drugs. *Amer. J. Psychiat.* 127 (1970):199–207.

219. Spiegel, D.E., Keith-Spiegel, P.: The effects of carphenazine, trifluoperazine and chlorpromazine on ward behavior, physiological functioning and psychological test scores in chronic schizophrenic patients. *J. Nerv. Ment. Dis.* 144 (1967:111–116.

220. Stallone, F., Shelley, E., Mendlewicz, J., Fieve, R.R.: The use of lithium in affective disorders, III: A double-blind study of prophylaxis in bipolar illness. *Amer. J. Psychiat.* 130 (1973):1006–1010.

221. Van Steenkiste, J.: La perphénazine, Indications. *Psychopharmacologie* Mars-Avril (Suppl. Encéphale) 60 (1971):63–70.

222. Strömgen, E.: Verlauf der Schizophrenien. In: *2. Weissenauer schizophreniesymposion, 4.+5.5.1973*, hsg. von Huber, G., pp. 121–136; F.K.Schattauer Verlag, Stuttgart-New York 1973.

223. Sutter, J.-M., Scotto, J.-C., Luccioni, H., Dufour, H., Alerini, P.: Essai contrôlé de la perphénazine dans le traitement des schizophrénies anciennes. *Encéphale* 60 (1971):136–164.

224. Swanson, D.W., Smith, J.A., Perez, H.: A fixed combination of chlorpromazine and trifluoperazine in psychotic patients. *Dis. Nerv. Syst.* 28 (1967):756.

225. Tanghe, A., Vereecken, J.L.T.M.: Fluspirilene, an injectable, and penfluridol, an oral, long-acting neuroleptic. A comparative double-blind trial in residual schizophrenia. *Acta Psychiat. Scand.* 48 (1972):315–331.

226. Temkov, I.: Home treatment of schizophrenics with long-acting major tranquillizers: social and psychological assessment. *Psychopharmacologia* (Berl.) 26, Suppl. (1972):108.

227. Turek, I.S., Ota, K.Y., Bohm, M., Kurland, A.A.: Piperacetazine vs. chlorpromazine in the treatment of schizophrenia. *Internat. Pharmacopsychiat.* (Basel) 4 (1970):239–244.

228. Turunen, S., Salminen, J.: Neuroleptic treatment and mortality. *Dis. Nerv. Syst.* 29 (1968):474–477.

229. Uhlir, F., Ryznar, J.: Appearance of chlorpromazine in the mother's milk. *Activ. Nerv. Sup.* (Prag) 15 (1973):106.

229a. Usdin, E., Efron, D.H.: Psychotropic drugs and related compounds, second edition, DHEW Publication No. (HSM):72–9074, Rockville, Maryland 1972.

230. Valzelli, L.: Psychopharmacology: An introduction to experimental and clinical principles. Essman, W.B., ed.; Spectrum Publications Halsted-Press, John Wiley & Sons, 1973.

231. Vojtechovsky, M.: Effects of treatment with lithium salts. In: *Problémy psychiatrie v praxi a ve výzkumu*, pp. 216–218; Praha 1957.

232. Vulpe, M.: Skin pigmentation and the phenothiazines. Neurological aspects. In: *Toxicity and adverse reaction studies with neuroleptics and antidepressants,* edit. by Lehmann, H.E., Ban, T.A., pp. 56–59; Quebec Psychopharmacological Research Ass., Verdun 1967.

233. Van Waes, A., Van de Velde: Safety evaluation of haloperidol in the treatment of hyperemesis gravidarum. *J. Clin. Pharmacol.* 9 (1969): 224–227.

234. Warner, H.: Skin pigmentation and the phenothiazines. Gastroenterological aspects. In: *Toxicity and adverse reaction studies with neuroleptics and antidepressants,* edit. by Lehmann, H.E., Ban, T.A., p. 70; Quebec Psychopharmacological Research Ass., Verdun 1967.

235. Waters, M.A., Northover, J.: Rehabilitated longstay schizophrenics in the community. *Brit. J. Psychiat.* 3 (1965):258–267.

236. Wendkos, M.H.: Electrocardiographic changes with psychoactive drugs. Experiments with thioridazine. In: *Toxicity and Adverse Reaction Studies with Neuroleptics and Antidepressants,* edited by Lehmann, H.E., Ban, T.A., 143–155; Quebec Psychopharmacological Research Ass., Verdun 1967.

237. Wessler, M.M., Kahn, V.L.: Can the chronic schizophrenic patient remain in the community? A follow-up study of twenty-four long-term hospitalized patients returned to the community. *J. Nerv. Ment. Dis.* 136 (1963):455–463.

238. Williams, J.R., Solecki, R.T., Puttkammer, S.: Effects of single, combined, and non-drug treatment on chronic mental patients (a preliminary study). *Dis. Nerv. Syst.* 30 (1969):696–701.

239. Wright, R.L.D., Lynes, P.G.: Value of continuous drug administration for chronic long-term mental hospital patients. *Canad. psychiat. Ass. J.* 9 (1964):352–357.

240. Youdim, M.B.H.: Significance of selective inhibition of multiple forms of monoamine oxidase. Collegium Internationale Neuropsycho-pharmacologicum, IX congr., Paris, 7–12/7/1974; symposia, abstracts in: *J Pharmacol.* 5/suppl. 1 (1974):99.

241. Zwanikren, G.J.: Penfluridol (R 16341). A long acting oral neuroleptic as maintenance therapy for schizophrenic and mentally retarded patients. A placebo controlled double blind trial. *Psychiat. Neurol. Neurochir.* (Amst.) 76 (1973):83–92.

INDEX OF GENERIC AND TRADE NAMES

INDEX OF SYNDROMES

Nathan S. Kline, M.D., is one of a handful of pioneers responsible for the introduction, in the early 1950s, of modern psychotropic drugs into clinical use in the United States. For this achievement, and for his role in the introduction, in 1956, of antidepressant medication in the treatment of psychiatric patients, he received, on two separate occasions, the Albert Lasker Clinical Research Award. Later he and his colleagues were to publish the first paper on the management of alcoholism through the use of lithium carbonate. He has in addition been prominently involved in the introduction and evaluation of at least a dozen other psychotropics, including many of the minor tranquilizers. Dr. Kline received his M.D. from the New York University College of Medicine and did his internship and residency at Saint Elizabeths Hospital in Washington, D.C. He was for a time Director of Research at Worcester State Hospital and is currently Director of the Rockland Research Institute, Clinical Professor of Psychiatry at Columbia University, Permanent Visiting Professor at the University of California at San Diego, and Medical Director of Regent Hospital, New York City.

Jules Angst, M.D., the distinguished Swiss psychiatrist and recipient of the Anna Monika Prize for research in depression, and the Paul Martini Prize, was granted his Doctorate in Medicine by the Medical Faculty of the University of Zurich, and the degree in psychiatry and psychotherapy of the Foederatio Medicorum Helveticorum. For many years Dr. Angst practiced at the Zurich Psychiatric University Hospital—the famous "Burgholzli"—advancing to the position, once held by Eugen Bleuler, of head physician for clinical psychiatry and psychology. He was for a time engaged in research at the Maudsley Hospital, London. Currently he is professor, research director, and head of the department of psychiatry at the University of Zurich and a member of many international professional societies.